SHOPPING IN 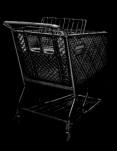 THE DARK?

WHAT IS HIDDEN IN YOUR SHOPPING CART?

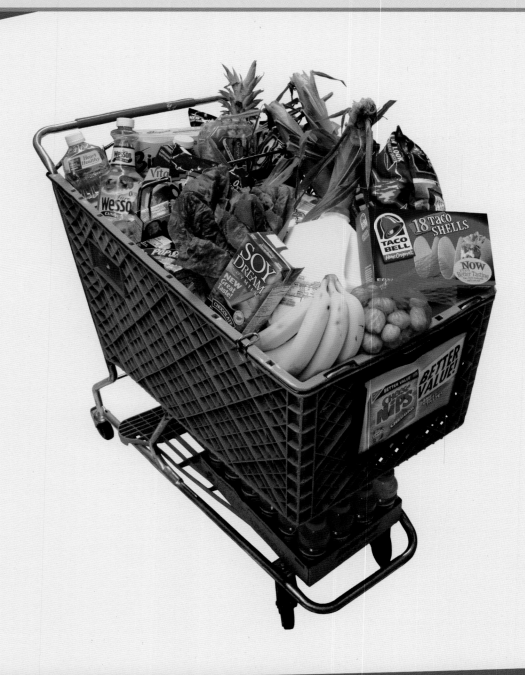

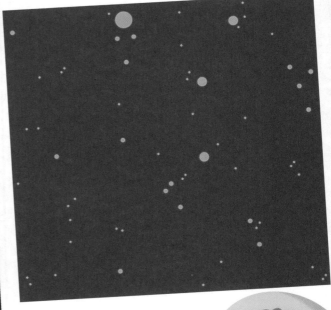

...015, a ...acecraft ...otured the ...st detailed ...otos of Pluto, ...luding an ...ea people call ...to's 'heart'!

 Pluto was discovered by an astronomer looking at photographs of the stars who saw that one faint 'star' was in different places in different photos — meaning it was orbiting the Sun. This was no star at all. It was Pluto! Spot the difference between these two pictures to discover Pluto for yourself.

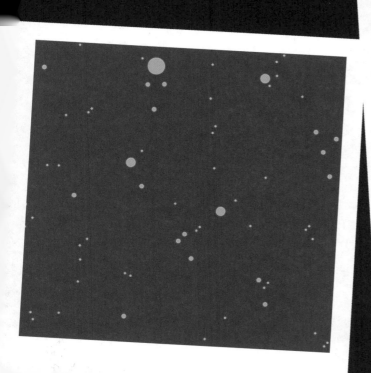

Hint: All the stars stay in the same place – Pluto is the only thing

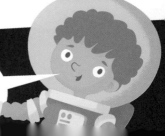

Dwarf planets

Around the Solar System there is a ring of millions of icy blocks, called the Kuiper Belt. The Kuiper Belt houses Pluto, as well as several more dwarf planets.

The planets are named after ancient Roman and Greek gods, but astronomers have run out of these names. The names of dwarf planets come from myths told all over the world, from Norway to the Pacific Ocean!

Dwarf planets
A dwarf planet is something big enough to form into a ball shape, but not big enough to push all the other space rocks out of its orbit. Only planets can do that.

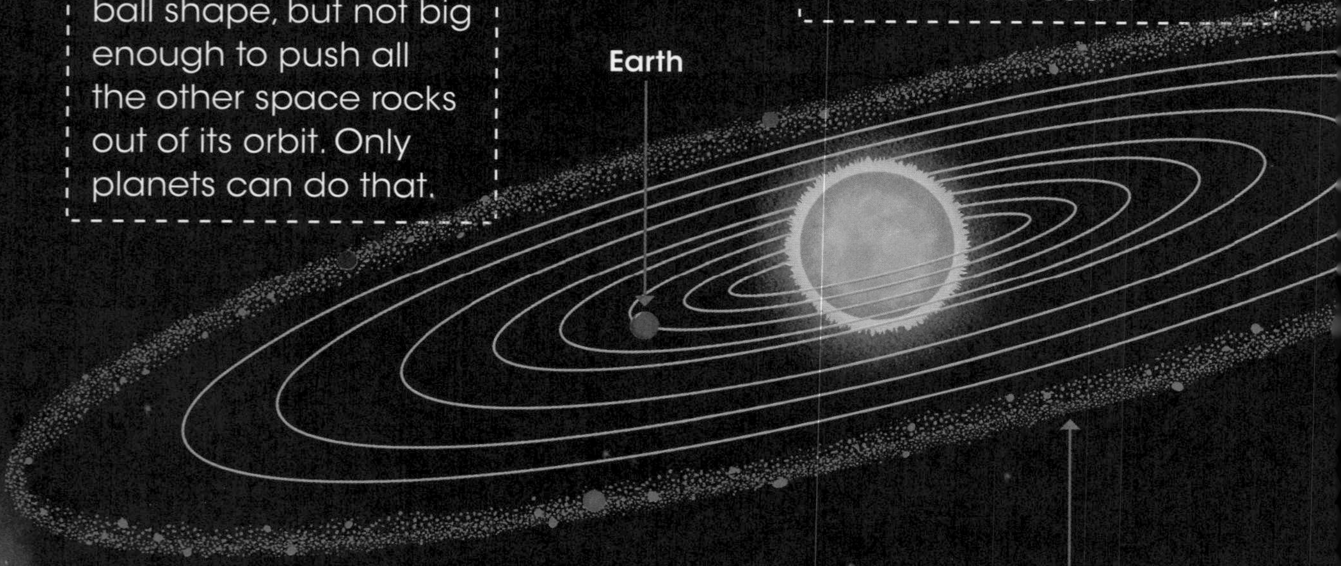

Earth

Kuiper Belt

We know of five dwarf planets, but astronomers think there must be many more.

Oort cloud
Beyond the Kuiper Belt there is an even larger cloud of icy chunks, called the Oort Cloud.

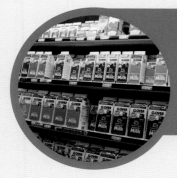

Beware of milk that has been produced using the genetically engineered hormone, rbGH. Thankfully, this hormone is outlawed from organic production.

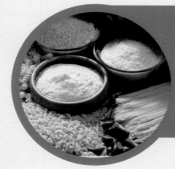

GE varieties of rice and wheat have been kept off the market by concerned citizens, farmers, and advocates. With continued vigilance, these crops will remain GE-free.

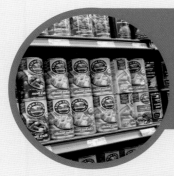

Danger! About 75% of processed foods contain at least one GE ingredient.

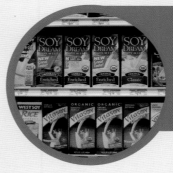

The USDA organic seal can steer you towards GE-free soy products. Without this seal, soy products are very likely to contain genetically engineered soybeans.

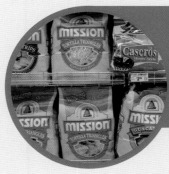

Watch out! Approximately 52% of corn grown in the U.S. is genetically engineered.

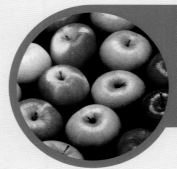

No worries here – the vast majority of fresh fruits and vegetables are grown without genetic engineering.

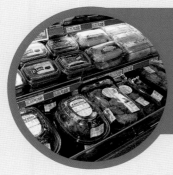

Currently no meat on the market has come from GE animals. However, unless they are certified organic, livestock may have been raised on genetically engineered grains.

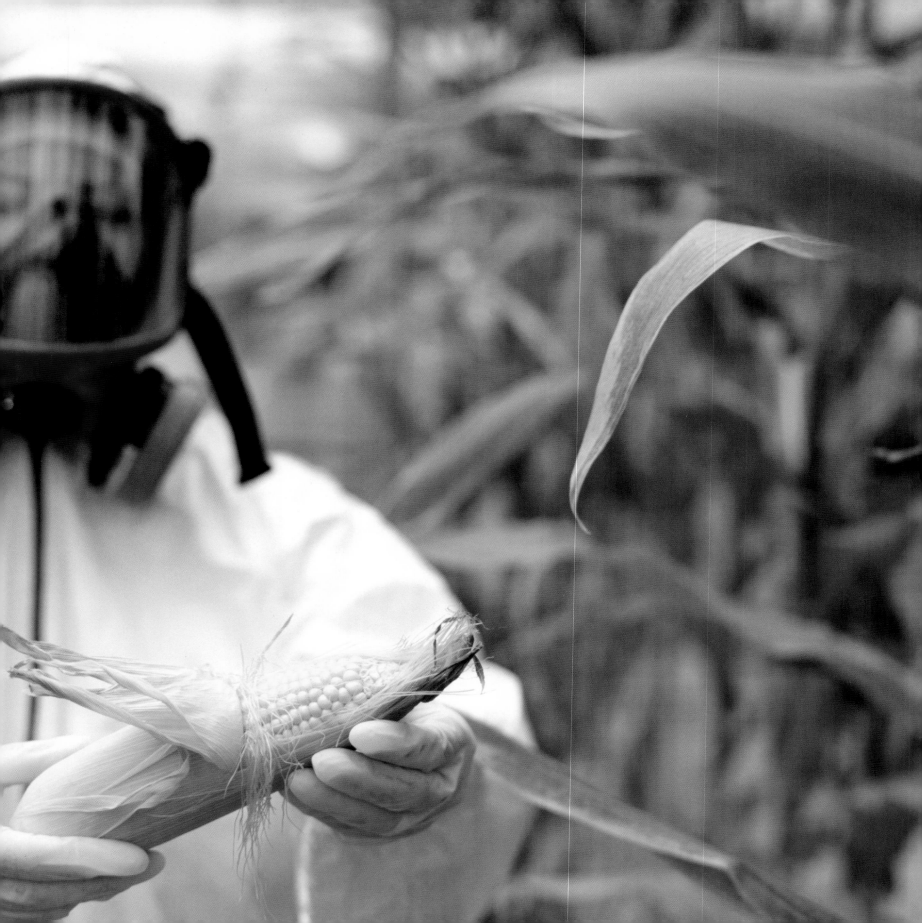

YOUR RIGHT

GENETIC ENGINEERING AND THE SECRET CHANGES IN YOUR FOOD

TO KNOW

"The children of North America have now become
the world's lab animals on whom to study
the long-term effects of eating GM products."[1]

—*Jane Goodall,*
Primatologist and author

Earth Aware Editions

17 Paul Drive

San Rafael, CA 94903

800.688.2218

www.earthawareeditions.com

Library of Congress Cataloging-in-Publication Data available.

ISBN 1-932771-19-0 paper
ISBN 1-932771-52-2 cloth

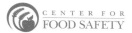

National Office:

660 Pennsylvania Avenue, SE

Suite 302

Washington, DC 20003

800.600.6664

www.centerforfoodsafety.org

West Coast Office:

2601 Mission Street

Suite 803

San Francisco, CA 94110

REPLANTED PAPER

Palace Press International, in association with Global ReLeaf, will plant two trees for
each tree used in the manufacturing of this book. Global ReLeaf is an international
campaign by American Forests, the nation's oldest nonprofit conservation organization
and a world leader in planting trees for environmental restoration.

americanforests.org
GLOBAL
RELEAF

10 9 8 7 6 5 4 3 2 1

Cover photograph © Xavier Bonghi / Getty Images

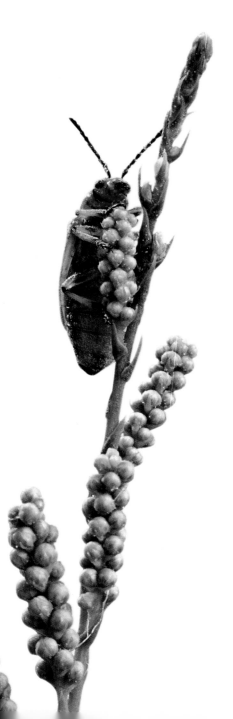

YOUR RIGHT

GENETIC ENGINEERING AND THE SECRET CHANGES IN YOUR FOOD

TO KNOW

Andrew Kimbrell
Center for Food Safety

Foreword by
Nell Newman

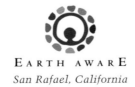

EARTH AWARE
San Rafael, California

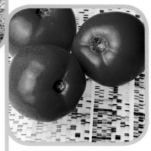

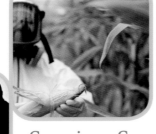

THREE

Sowing Seeds of Destruction......56

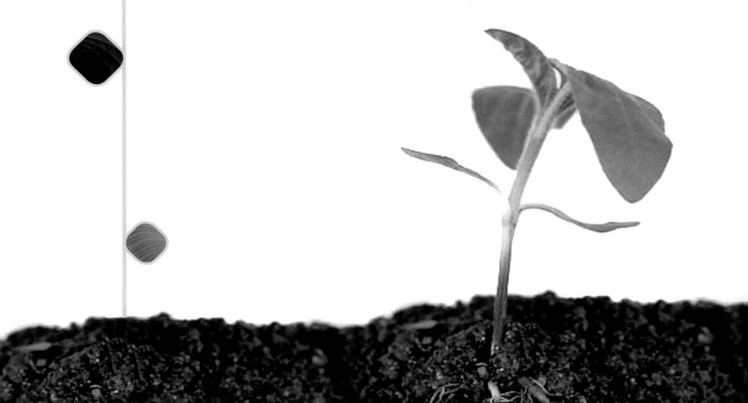

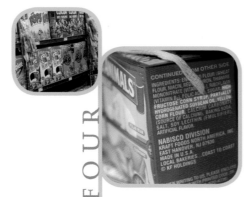

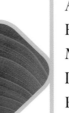

FOUR

A Quick Guide to Genetically Engineered Foods in Your Supermarket......78

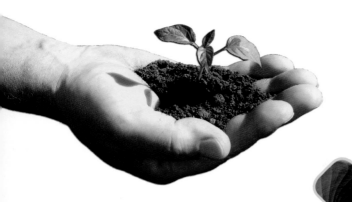

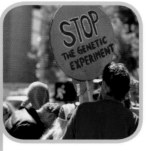

Choosing the Future of Food......*94*

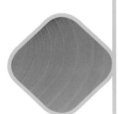

APPENDICES......*118*

FIVE

Foreword

Nell Newman

NELL NEWMAN
is co-founder and president
of Newman's Own Organ-
ics, a food company producing
products including snack foods,
cookies, oils, pet foods, and
more. The daughter of ac-
tors Paul Newman and Joanne
Woodward, Nell had an early
introduction to natural foods. At
their rural Connecticut home,
the family had a garden and
raised chickens, and Nell was
taught to cook by her mother,
as well as spending many hours
fishing with her father. Nell
attended the College of the
Atlantic in Bar Harbor, Maine,
graduating with a B.S. in human
ecology. She worked briefly
at the Environmental Defense
Fund in New York, but, prefer-
ring a more rural environment,
moved to Northern California. She held a position at the
Ventana Wilderness Sanctuary,
which was working to reestab-
lish the bald eagle in central
California. After two and a half
years, she left Ventana Wilderness Sanctuary and began
fundraising for the Santa Cruz
Predatory Bird Research Group.
In 1993, she founded Newman's
Own Organics, a division of
Newman's Own.

Food has been my work and passion for many years now. During that time, I, along with so many others, have devoted myself to ensuring a safe and sustainable food future for succeeding generations.
Unfortunately, many in agribusiness still stand in the way of that food future as they promote the arti-
ficial-is-better view of food production. They dream of a completely industrialized food supply—one
wholly dependent on pesticides, other toxic chemicals, and a brew of artificial additives—that threatens our health and the natural world. Meanwhile, the organic movement is working to realize a very
different vision of food production, one committed to the most natural, sustainable, healthy, and tasty
food supply possible.

The problem of genetically engineered (GE) foods is at the heart of this historic struggle,
causing confusion and concern among millions of Americans. When I'm asked about these novel foods
—as I am with increasing frequency — my first response comes from my background as a biologist. It's
clear to me that a handful of chemical corporations have rushed gene-altered foods into our fields and
supermarkets without conducting the science needed to demonstrate the safety of these foods for our
children, the environment, and us. In fact, independent studies coming in from universities and government agencies, both here and abroad, demonstrate the hazards that these biotech foods can present
to our health and to the natural world.

Even as these disturbing results are reported, the Food and Drug Administration (FDA)
neither requires the biotechnology industry to conduct studies on the potential toxicity or allergenicity
or nutritional value of these foods, nor do they mandate ecological research on the contamination of
other crops and the destruction of ecosystems and wildlife. To make matters worse, the U.S. is virtually
alone in failing to demand the labeling of genetically engineered foods among the leading agricultural
nations, despite the fact that polls consistently show that more than 90 percent of Americans want
these foods identified. Without adequate science and labeling, we are all eating in the dark: We don't
know what genetically engineered material is in our food or what those foods are doing to us and to
our families. We have become unwilling guinea pigs in a vast biological experiment with our food.
Genetic engineering is not only a serious public-health issue, but a real challenge to the very concept of
government of, by, and for the people.

My profound concern about the effects of genetic engineering in our food and on our democracy is matched by my deep dismay over its dire impact on organic agriculture. To put it bluntly, I
join thousands of other organic growers and producers who are outraged by extensive plantings of GE
crops in the U.S. These crops threaten our livelihood and the future of the entire organics industry.
And though organics continue to be the fastest-growing agricultural sector in America, the practice of
genetic engineering represents the single-greatest danger to the future of organic food. Meanwhile, a
few biotechnology corporations and their friends in government imperil all the good work done by so

many in the organic movement over the last several decades.

Biotech foods jeopardize organics in two ways. The first is through genetic contamination. New genes engineered into foods by Monsanto and other GE-food companies can and have escaped from plants—via wind, insects, rain, and other sources—and crossed into conventionally and organically grown crops. Both national and international standards forbid the use of genetic engineering in any foods labeled "organic," meaning the products of these contaminated crops and seeds cannot be sold as organic.

Unfortunately, this is not just a theoretical possibility. At present, four crops—corn, soy, canola, and cotton—have been genetically engineered and commercialized, and we have seen biological pollution of crops and plants from all these GE varieties. Organic corn seed, for instance, is increasingly difficult and expensive to find and buy because GE varieties have contaminated virtually all supplies. If crops like wheat, rice, and a slew of fruits and vegetables are engineered, and the results are marketed in the U.S., the growth of the organic sector will be seriously hampered—indeed, the very existence of organic food could be threatened.

The second assault by GE foods on organic agriculture is subtler, but potentially as fatal. Close to 20 percent of GE crops planted in this country contain a manipulated genetic construct of the natural, non-chemical pesticide Bacillus thuringiensis (Bt). Bt, instead of traditional pesticides, is one of the few options organic farmers have to control pests. As millions of acres of crops are planted with gene-altered Bt, resistance to it is built up in insects, making Bt ineffective in controlling them. This robs organic farmers of their major tool for containing pests, forcing potentially thousands of growers back to using chemical inputs—and out of organic farming.

Whether you are part of the organic movement, as I am, or just an interested member of the public, *Your Right to Know: Genetic Engineering and the Secret Changes in Your Food* is a must-read on this vitally important food issue. The scientists, food experts, farmers, and health professionals who have come together to produce this book do us all a real service. They have presented an informative, well-researched, accessible, and yes, even entertaining primer on everything we need to know about these foods, and smart, consumer-friendly ways to avoid them. This book shines a bright light on the GE foods controversy, defeating the attempt of the biotech industry and those in government who keep us forever in the dark about the environmental, social and human health consequences of GE foods. I invite you to read the following pages carefully—and to join us in the fight for a new, organic food future.

"The Food and Drug Administration (FDA) neither requires the biotechnology industry to conduct studies on the potential toxicity or allergenicity or nutritional value of these foods, nor do they mandate ecological research on the contamination of other crops and the destruction of ecosystems and wildlife."

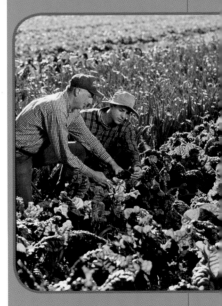

Introduction

Andrew Kimbrell

ANDREW KIMBRELL is founder and executive director of the Washington D.C.-based Center for Food Safety and the International Center for Technology Assessment. As an author, lawyer, and activist for more than twenty years, Andrew has been at the forefront of legal and grassroots efforts o protect the environment and promote sustainable agricultural production methods. He edited *Fatal Harvest: The Tragedy of Industrial Agriculture* and *The Green Lifestyle Handbook* and wrote *The Human Body Shop: The Engineering and Marketing of Life* and *The Masculine Mystique: Men and Technology*. Andrew has been featured on radio and television programs across the country, including the *Today Show*, *The Early Show*, *Crossfire*, and *Good Morning America*. His written work has appeared in numerous newspapers and magazines including *The New York Times*, *Washington Post*, and *Harper's*. He has lectured at dozens of universities throughout the country and has testified at numerous congressional and regulatory hearings. In 1994, the *Utne Reader* named Kimbrell as one of the world's leading 100 visionaries.

The genetic engineering of our food may well be the most profound alteration in our diet since the advent of agriculture ten thousand years ago. In the past, our ancestors selected from naturally occurring variations to gradually transform wild plants into food crops more suitable for the human population. Seeds were then seen as the common heritage of humanity and generally available for saving, storage, and dissemination.

Now a handful of transnational companies have used relatively crude biotechnology techniques to engineer foreign genetic material into many of our staple crops. Ignoring millennia of evolution and selective breeding, they have added, among other novel genetic material, viral, pesticidal, and antibiotic resistance genes into every cell of these plants. In this way, new and potentially harmful substances never before seen in plants end up in our fields and in the foods we eat. These same corporations have also placed patents on these plants and the techniques used to transform them, giving them monopoly control of the seeds.

Many Americans are understandably confused and anxious about the presence of these genetically engineered (GE) foods on our supermarket shelves. With an estimated 70 to 75 percent of processed foods now containing genetically engineered ingredients, the public feels it has a right to know about the presence of genetically modified foods in their diets. Polls consistently show that up to 90 percent of Americans want these genetically engineered foods labeled. Despite this clear public mandate for choice, our Food and Drug Administration (FDA) has for more than a decade continued its policy of not requiring the labeling or human health testing of these foods. In fact, the FDA has completely ignored the public interest and, at the behest of the biotechnology industry, refused to establish any mandatory regulations whatsoever on GE foods. Meanwhile, governments throughout Europe and the world are requiring strict labeling and testing of these foods and some are rejecting them outright.

As our FDA continues its misguided and isolated policy of not testing or labeling of genetically engineered foods, the public has been left to "eat in the dark." Not willing to be unwitting guinea pigs in this vast food experiment, the public urgently needs more information about these novel foods and answers to some critical questions:

- Are these genetically engineered foods safe for my family and me?
- Do they harm the environment?
- What is their impact on our traditional crops?
- How do these genetically engineered plants and the corporate patents on them affect our farmers and the farm community?

In this book, the Center for Food Safety provides information you can trust and straightforward answers to these important concerns and many other questions about this controversial new food technology. We have used the most up-to-date scientific information to look behind the corporate and media hype about these foods and reveal the facts about their impacts. In Chapter 1, we use numerous scientific studies and the findings of U.S. government scientists to describe and explain the health risks of GE foods. In Chapter 2, we explain the increasing evidence and concern about how growing these foods can affect our natural environment and contaminate non-GE crops. In Chapter 3, we examine how the introduction of these crops is affecting farmers and our already beleaguered farm communities.

Even as we provide you with this information, we understand that perhaps the most important question that the public has about GE foods is about choice:

- Since our government has refused to label these foods, how do we avoid buying and eating these foods?

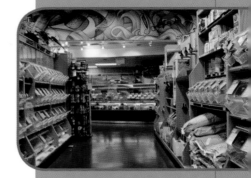

Chapter 4 of this book is a uniquely designed shopper's guide on GE foods. We take you through each section of the supermarket and explain how to identify foods with genetically engineered ingredients. This is not a confusing list of hundreds of products and product names that you will have to remember or carry around with you. Rather, it provides the reader with simple, user-friendly, yet effective principles and tips that will empower you to identify where GE ingredients are in your supermarket and thereby allow you to choose not to buy or consume them. For those who want more in-depth information, in the book's appendix, we provide a more detailed product listing. We also understand that even as many in the public would like to avoid these foods in the supermarket or eating out, they would also like to get more involved in this important issue about our collective food future. Chapter 5 of this book describes how you can get active at the local, state, and even federal levels to ensure that your right to know about the food you and your family eat is respected and protected. Here you will read of many people throughout the country who have, often successfully, challenged corporate and government power on this important issue.

Throughout, we have gone to great lengths to ensure that this book is as accurate and up-to-date as possible. But clearly, more scientific evidence is constantly coming in and corporations and governments do change their policies. Therefore, we have provided a list of phone numbers and websites of corporations, government agencies, and advocacy organizations that will help you keep up with new developments. Additionally, the CFS website (www.centerforfoodsafety.org) will have a specific link that updates this book periodically. The book also provides a reading list for those who wish to further explore the scientific and policy issues related to this technology.

We hope this book becomes an important tool ensuring your right to know. Please read it carefully and share it with family and friends. Together we can create a healthy, humane, and sustainable food future.

"Now a handful of transnational companies have used relatively crude biotechnology techniques to engineer foreign genetic material into many of our staple crops. Ignoring millennia of evolution and selective breeding, they have added, among other novel genetic material, viral, pesticidal, and antibiotic resistance genes into every cell of these plants. In this way, new and potentially harmful substances never before seen in plants end up in our fields and in the foods we eat."

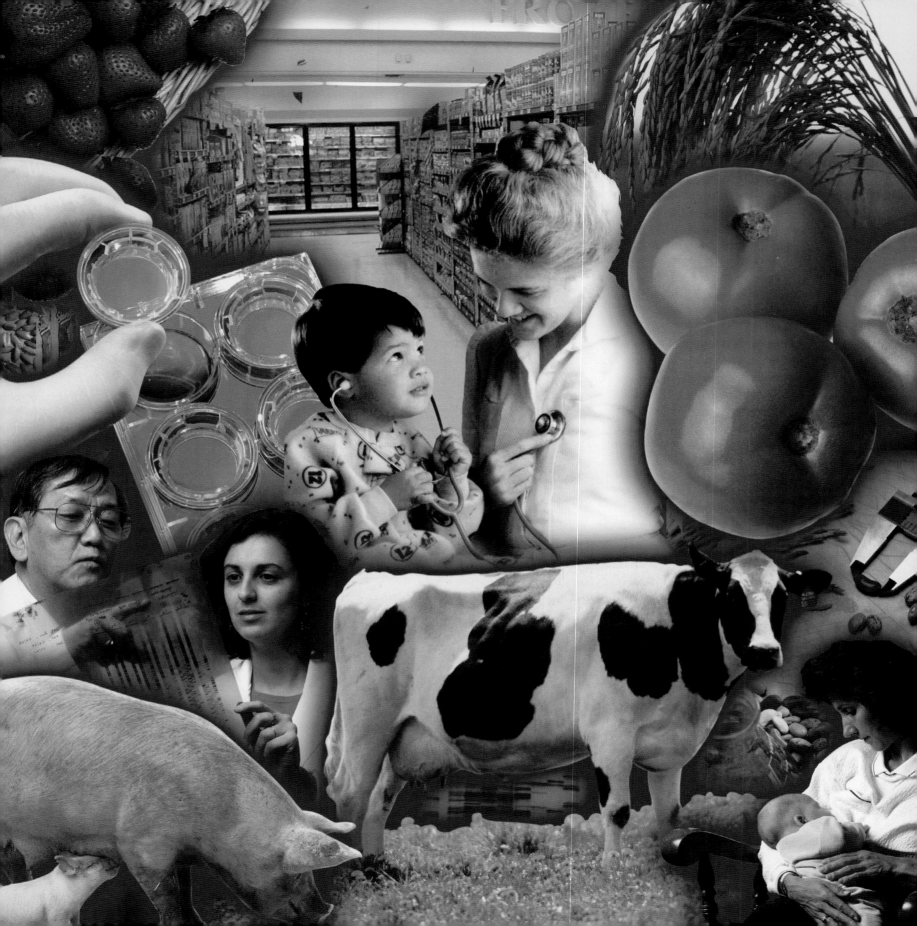

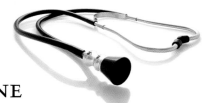

CHAPTER ONE

The Real Human Health Risks

a Pediatrician speaks out

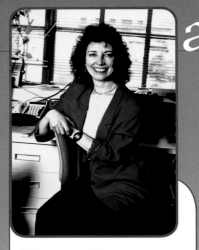

MARTHA HERBERT, M.D., PH.D. is a pediatric neurologist associated with Massachusetts General Hospital, Cambridge Health Alliance, and Harvard Medical School. She specializes in learning and developmental disorders and researches brain structure in children with autism. She received her medical degree from Columbia University College of Physicians and Surgeons, her pediatrics training at New York Hospital-Cornell University Medical Center, and her neurology training at the Massachusetts General Hospital. Herbert also works on health and ecological risks of genetically modified food and on neurotoxins and brain development. Prior to her medical training she obtained an interdisciplinary doctorate from the History of Consciousness program at UC Santa Cruz, studying evolution and development of learning processes in biology and culture.

MARTHA HERBERT, M.D., PH.D. TELLS WHY SHE'S CONCERNED ABOUT GE FOODS.

Q: Why do you call genetically modified food "one of the largest uncontrolled experiments in modern history"?

In medicine, we expect to be informed about participating in experiments and given the right to consent or to refuse to participate. It's considered unethical and illegal for the medical profession to experiment on you without your informed consent. But no such standards apply in our food supply. Certain companies have flooded the marketplace with thousands of untested food products containing foreign genetic material with no label to alert us to these ingredients. The health effects have not been seriously studied. That means consumers are unknowingly test subjects.

Q: What harm can genetically modified food do to people?

Genes from other species engineered into food products make proteins that normally aren't made by that type of food. These proteins are mostly intended to retard spoilage, fight off insects, or protect the plant against pesticides. Most of these proteins are not there to make food more nutritious. Could these proteins be toxic? Could they challenge the immune system? Could they damage a baby's developing nervous system? Could they cause problems in people with chronic illness? The right studies have not been done to find out. Genetically modified foods could cause big problems like serious allergies, or they could cause nagging and annoying problems like bowel or stomach discomfort or skin rashes that could be hard to trace to these foods.

Q: What do parents need to know?

Infants' intestinal barrier functions and immune systems are not fully developed. This is why pediatricians are careful about introducing new proteins into infant diets. Without labeling, parents have no way of knowing whether or not the soy formula they're feeding their babies contains untested proteins. There is a lot of evidence that food can affect health. Early diet can be related to later diseases. The doubling of childhood asthma since 1980 has been linked to early diet. Certain foods can trigger behavior changes in vulnerable children such as some with autism or attention deficit disorder. All parents—but especially the parents of the many babies with colic, food intolerance, or diseases or chronic health problems of any kind—should be able to make choices about the ingredients in their children's food.

Q: Who's testing and tracking health impacts of genetically modified food products?

Nobody. Companies that sell genetically modified products aren't required to conduct thorough health studies before putting their products on the market. And there is no monitoring system in place. Tracking the millions of people with vulnerable immune systems and their reaction to novel proteins and virus fragments in genetically modified food is impossible without food labeling. This means that our public health system isn't taking these risks seriously. This isn't sound science, and it isn't sound public health practice.

Q: Is the Food and Drug Administration (FDA) right to say genetically modified products are just like those made the old-fashioned way?

Chicken genes in apples? Fish genes in strawberries? That's never been done before. Apples with chicken genes or strawberries with fish genes may have different levels of nutrients that could affect health. People with chicken or fish allergies might react from eating these apples or strawberries, and without labels they would have no idea why. Also, the methods used to insert these genes can disrupt essential genetic function, changing which genes get turned on or how much they do. But genetically engineered foods aren't systematically tested for these kinds of changes.

Q: Can genetically modified foods make antibiotics less effective?

Genes for antibiotic resistance are used as markers to test the success of attempted gene transfers—basically, for corporate convenience. If you attach these markers to the foreign gene you're sticking into the food and then dump lots of antibiotic on the food, you know you engineered the gene into the food cells if the food is not harmed by the antibiotic. But then, if your body or your normal gut bacteria take up these antibiotic resistance genes, common antibiotics like ampicillin might not help when you're sick.

Q: How can the government protect us?

If we're going to have genetically modified food, any food with genetically modified material should be clearly labeled so the consumer knows. We need complete, thorough, long-term, independent evaluation of these novel organisms before they're produced or sold. Better yet, if we don't have consensus that all the necessary tests have been done on these foods, we should not be growing and eating genetically modified organisms. As pediatricians often tell parents, and parents often tell kids: "Better safe than sorry."

WHAT DO AMERICANS WANT?

Recent opinion polls[1] show consistently that an overwhelming majority of Americans—up to 90 percent—support the labeling of GE foods. Close to 60 percent would avoid such foods if they were identified. Clearly, the public wants GE foods to be marked, yet our government still refuses to listen to those it purports to represent.

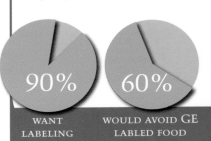

90%
WANT LABELING

60%
WOULD AVOID GE LABLED FOOD

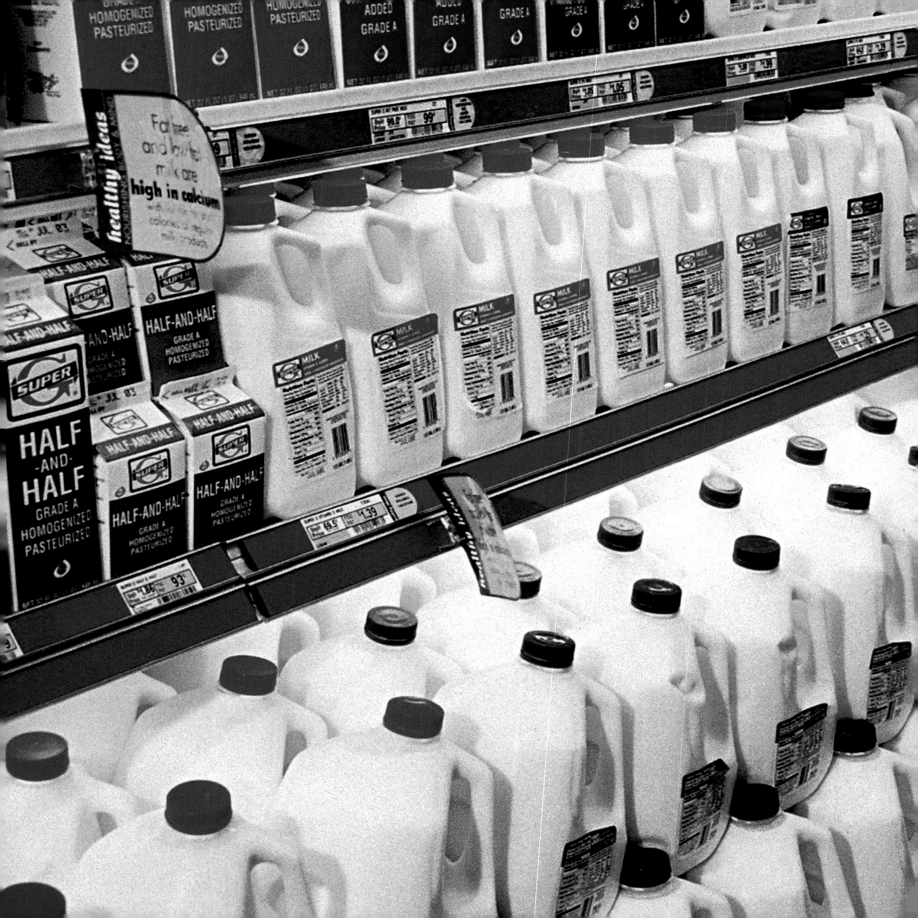

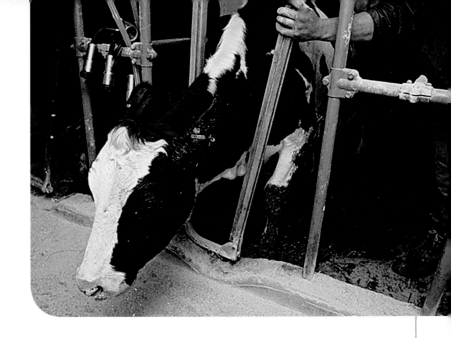

GOT HORMONES?

MANY AMERICANS FIRST HEARD about the possible genetic engineering of our food supply in the mid-1980s. At that time, Monsanto and three other biotech companies were developing a genetically engineered (GE) hormone, recombinant bovine growth hormone (rbGH), to inject into cows to enable them to produce more milk. Monsanto spent hundreds of millions of dollars developing rbGH for commercial use and hyping it as a new miracle technology to increase milk supply.

Long before it was approved by the Food and Drug Administration (FDA) in 1994, rbGH sparked controversy among farming, food safety, and animal-welfare advocates. At the outset, critics noted that the U.S. was already awash in milk and spending millions of tax dollars to destroy cows and reduce its production.[2] The significant but unneeded increase in milk production—Monsanto predicted a 25 percent gain—would hurt small-scale dairy farmers and their communities by lowering milk prices. The winners would be the large-scale farm conglomerates that could absorb the cost.

Soon, immediate threats to consumers came to light. The first involved a hormone called "insulin-like growth factor-1" (IGF-1). Milk from rbGH-treated cows,

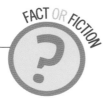

"Genetic Engineering—of food and other products—has far outrun the science that must be its first governing discipline. Therein lie the peril, the risk, and the foolhardiness... the wanton release of genetically engineered products is tantamount to flying blind."[4]

—*Ralph Nader*

according to Monsanto's own figures reported to the FDA, contains higher levels of IGF-1 than milk from untreated cows.[5] Scientific research has shown that IFG-1-tainted milk survives the human digestion process and ends up in our bodies.[6] The problem? Negative health risks. A 1995 conference at the National Institutes of Health (NIH) identified the following potential adverse effects of IGF-1:[7]

1. Strong role in breast cancer

2. Special risk of colon cancer due to local effects on the gastrointestinal tract

3. A possible role in osteosarcoma, the most common bone cancer in children, usually occurring during the adolescent growth spurt

4. Implicated in lung cancer

More recently, studies conducted by Harvard Medical School and other institutions confirm the FDA's fears: Elevated levels of IGF-1 in the body are linked to a higher risk of colon, prostate, and breast cancers.[8] Monsanto's rbGH has also been blamed for the massive suffering of livestock. Among other health impacts, the drug compounds the rate of painful and potentially fatal lameness in cows, causes major reproductive problems including mutations in offspring, and increases levels of mastitis, a painful udder infection.[9] Sick cows do not make wholesome milk, and the suffering caused by rbGH affects consumers' health, too. Food-safety experts note that rampant mastitis

forces farmers to use more antibiotics, thereby contaminating the cow's milk and reaching the milk-drinking public.[10] Furthermore, milk spoils faster because of higher somatic cell counts—more pus in the milk—from the diseased animals. Even worse, rbGH makes cattle more susceptible to "mad cow disease" by exposing the cow to greater amounts of potentially contaminated feed. And don't forget the risks of increased levels of IGF-1, discussed above.

Consumers were understandably upset about a product that threatened to add antibiotics, hormones, and pus to their milk while harming animals, increasing the potential for mad cow disease and destroying small-dairy farms. It looked like the only profit-makers would be Monsanto and large, factory-farm-type dairies.

The devastating health impacts of rbGH on cows prompted Canada, the European Union, and virtually every country around the world to ban its use. The suffering of animals alone is enough cause for consumers to avoid rbGH-derived dairy and meat products. The international regulators, including representatives from Canada and Europe, also shared concerns about the effects of rbGH on human health.[11]

Given the hormone's risks to cows and humans, and its rejection by the global agriculture community, how in the world did this drug get approved by our FDA?

It's an all-too-typical story of corporate influence on our government. In 1992, Michael Taylor went directly from working as an attorney on Monsanto's behalf to becoming the FDA's food policy deputy commissioner. Under his watch, rbGH was approved and its risks virtually ignored. Even worse, the agency failed to mandate the labeling of rbGH-derived products. Later, Taylor left the government and ran Monsanto's Washington, D.C. office. (See sidebar in Chapter 3, "What Is the Revolving Door?")

And yet, the FDA's chicanery couldn't save rbGH. The other three companies that were developing the drug dropped it, and despite huge financial and political pressure by Monsanto, rbGH remains banned in most of the world. In another blow to the drug, Monsanto had to suspend approximately 50 percent of all production and sale of the genetically engineered hormone in 2004 because of contamination.[13] One more thing Monsanto probably did not count on was consumers' strong rejection of rbGH. According to Datamonitor, which tracks supermarket sales, "growth in demand for organic milk is largely driven by the continued use of growth hormones such as rbGH and antibiotics in the conventional dairy industry."[14]

During its early days, rbGH was touted as the flagship food-production innovation of biotechnology. In many ways, the history of this hormone reveals important themes, repeated again and again, by companies that attempt to genetically engineer our food supply:

Human health threats. Genetic engineering presents dire risks to human health, but our government refuses to acknowledge or test these concerns.

Corporate influence. Genetically engineered foods were approved only after Monsanto and other corporate lawyers and scientists infiltrated our government agencies.

Taking away our choice. The FDA not only approved these gene-altered foods and products for sale, but also refused to mandate labeling for them, thereby depriving us of our right to know about these potentially hazardous foods.

Junk science. The FDA and other agencies either required no scientific evidence of the safety of biotech products or accepted uncritically the self-serving "junk" science that the biotech corporations gave them.

International isolation. As with rbGH, much of the world has rejected the U.S. approach and either banned genetically engineered products or demanded mandatory labeling and testing.

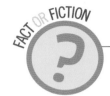

FACT OR FICTION
?

Genetic engineering is adding vitamins to our food.

Fiction There are no GE crops on the market with increased vitamin content. On the contrary, the FDA's own scientists warned that genetic engineering may decrease the nutritional content of our food.[15]

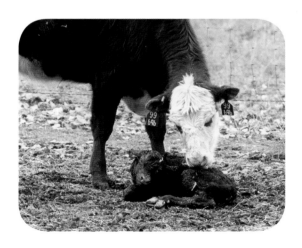
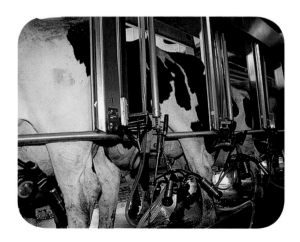
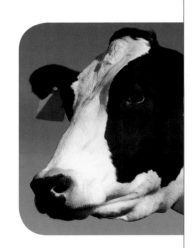

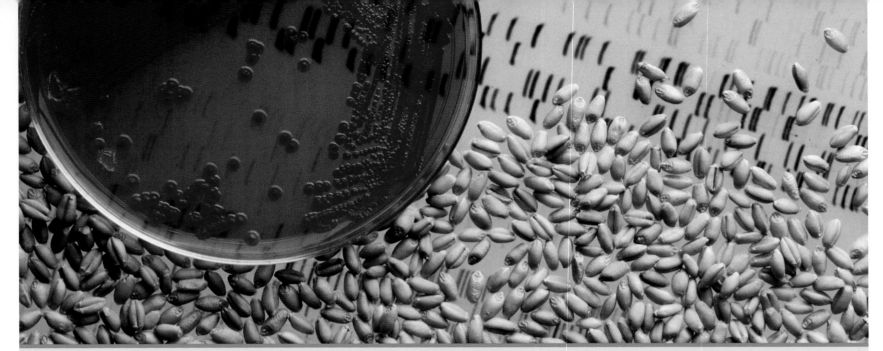

WHAT IS GENETIC ENGINEERING?

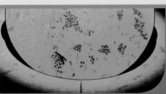

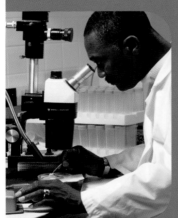

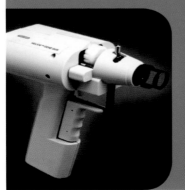

So how do genetic engineers get those flounder genes into tomatoes? They face a number of obstacles. The initial challenge is to invade the plant cell and deposit the desired new genes inside. One crude solution to this problem is the gene gun, a device that literally shoots the new genetic material into the cells. Slightly more subtle is the currently favored solution, which is to attach the gene to a vector capable of cell invasion. The best candidates for this task are, not surprisingly, vectors from bacteria and viruses. Most plant biotechnology relies on a bacterium to carry the foreign genetic construct into the cell.

Plant cells often reject alien genetic invaders altogether, and even when invasion does occur, other difficulties remain. When a gene comes from a different genetic context, plant cells may not be able to recognize the foreign gene to turn it on. To resolve this problem, viral promoters are often added to activate and promote the foreign gene. Whereas most of a plant's genes are turned on only in certain parts of a plant and at defined intervals during growth, viral promoters tend to turn on the new gene in virtually all parts of the plant during most stages of growth.[16]

As the gene inside the cell operates with an effective promoter, a final problem remains. In the midst of this hit-or-miss endeavor, how do the scientists know they have triumphed? To ascertain their success, biotech food producers call upon a marker gene that they inserted in the beginning, along with the gene of interest and the promoter. If active, the marker gene will render the cell impervious to a particular chemical, often an antibiotic or herbicide. Later, the plant tissue is flooded with the chemical, and if any cells survive, the scientists know that the genetic cassette has been integrated successfully into those cells.

Thus, genetic engineering is anything but a smooth, predictable operation. It is not a single, new gene that is cleanly inserted into a cell, but an entire cassette—usually the bacterial vector, the gene of interest, the viral promoters, and the marker system. And further, this cassette does not even insert into a specific place in the plant's genome. Instead, it is randomly introduced with the potential to disrupt other important plant functions. Each part in this process brings with it potential health threats to consumers.

OF FISH TOMATOES AND HUMAN PIGS

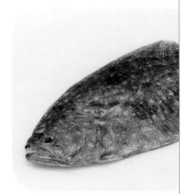

A round the same time Taylor and his co-horts at the FDA approved rbGH, they published a policy that allowed the marketing of GE foods without mandatory testing and labeling. Although they claimed that these foods were substantially the same as conventional foods, their statements were wrong and they knew it. The proponents of genetic engineering comprehended the ability of this new method to cross nature's barriers in ways never before imagined. Subsequently, biotech researchers have shattered species boundaries at will. Engineering human growth genes into fish, pigs, and other livestock to make them grow larger and more quickly; mixing flounder genes into tomatoes so they can grow and be stored at lower temperatures; adding pesticide genes into corn and other vegetables to resist pests; and even combining firefly genes with tobacco, causing the plants to glow twenty-four hours a day, for seemingly no purpose at all, are just a few of these experiments.

This mixing and matching of genetic material challenges the integrity of life on earth. It's not surprising that genetically engineered foods are profoundly different than other foods and present very unique risks to farm-ecology.

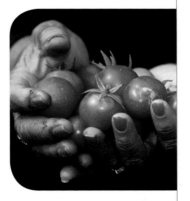

For the first time ever, foreign genes are in every cell of many of the foods we eat. (See sidebar: What Is Genetic Engineering?)

When the political appointees at the FDA ignored these facts and approved new genetically engineered plants without labeling or testing them, longtime scientists at the agency revolted. One scientist asked, "What happened to the scientific elements in [the] document?"[17] Another noted, "The processes of genetic engineering and traditional breeding are different, and according to the technical experts in the agency, they lead to different risks."[18] Yet another was even more blunt, saying, "We believe that animal feeds derived from genetically modified (GM) plants present unique animal and food safety concerns."[19]

Scientists issued a dire warning: These new, gene-engineered plants could cause serious allergies, render formerly non-toxic food toxic, increase our resistance to antibiotics, depress our immune systems, and remove the nutrition from our foods. In the rest of this chapter, we'll take a look at each of these important concerns.

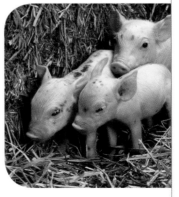

DISTRIBUTION OF GE CROPS WORLDWIDE*

United States: 55.3%   Canada: 6.4%

Argentina: 19.0%   China: 3.7%

  Brazil: 6.4%   All other countries: 5.2%

*Data from: James, C. 2005. Global Status of Commercialized Biotech/GM Crops: 2005. ISAAA Briefs No. 34. ISAA Ithaca, NY.

ALLERGIC REACTIONS

"I personally have no wish to eat anything produced by genetic modification, nor do I knowingly offer this sort of produce to my family or guests... We simply do not know the long-term consequences for human health and the wider environment." [20]

—*Charles, H.R.H. Prince of Wales*

Do you know what foods you react to? One out of four people in the U.S. reports having some type of food allergy.[21] Genetically engineered ingredients make matters worse in two ways.

First, shuffling genes among species causes an allergen, for example a nut allergen, to end up in food we've always thought is safe. Take what happened in 1996 when university researchers decided to check out a new genetically engineered soybean created by the Pioneer Hi-Bred International. The soybeans were engineered to contain a single gene from a Brazil nut. Since it's well known in the medical community that nuts can cause allergic reactions in people, the scientist decided to find out whether or not this single gene in the soybeans could cause a response in folks who were allergic to Brazil nuts. Incredibly, allergic reactions did occur from this one gene, as reported that year in the *New England Journal of Medicine*.[22] For people who are fatally allergic to Brazil nuts, eating this genetically engineered soy could be lethal. It's important to remember that this allergy test was done independently and at the discretion of these scientists; it was not required by any regulatory agency of the U.S.

The second danger is that genetically engineering foods can provoke an entirely new set of allergies. Here's how it works: The genetic packages transferred into the cell encode a number of novel proteins unfamiliar to the host plant. The resulting combination of a foreign gene and the genetic material of the plant can set off an allergic reaction. For example, in November 2005, Australian researchers found that peas, genetically engineered with a bean gene, triggered allergic reactions in research animals.[23] This was a surprise because the new gene in the peas was for a protein found in beans that does not cause any allergic reactions at all. How could these identical genes, one causing no allergies and the other causing allergies when engineered into a pea, have such a different impact? The same gene can produce slight variations of proteins in different plants—even in closely related plants. In the pea, the protein encoded by the gene was modified in a slightly different way than in the bean, and the new form of this protein was allergenic. So even when working with identical genes, the very process of genetic engineering can turn a non-allergenic gene into an allergenic one—a frightening prospect. Yet, this new finding should not come as a surprise. More than a decade ago, FDA scientists warned repeatedly that genetic engineering could "produce a new protein allergen," and they've demanded long-term testing for this hazard. Meanwhile, leaders at the FDA continue to ignore science and refuse to require solid testing of genetically engineered foods, exposing the public to these new and hidden allergens.

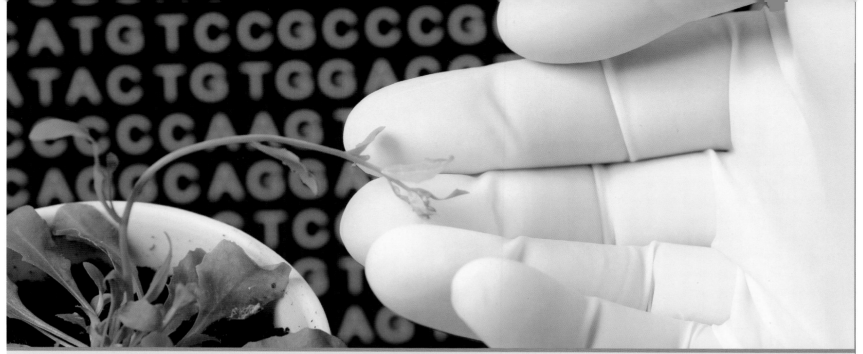

YOUR TAX DOLLARS (NOT) AT WORK

What the FDA does—and doesn't do—about GE foods.

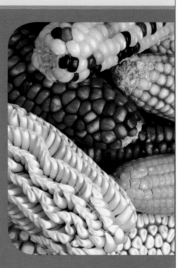

The Food and Drug Administration regulates the introduction of new foods and food additives and oversees labeling requirements. The FDA has the authority to remove unsafe foods from grocery shelves and hold companies accountable for the safety of their products. The agency can also require the pre-market approval of food additives, unless they are "generally regarded as safe" (GRAS). In 1992, the FDA declared genetically modified foods as substantially equivalent to conventional foods, deeming these new foods GRAS. This policy exempts GE foods from mandatory human and environmental safety tests and exempts them from labeling for their GE status.

The determination of substantial equivalence was ascertained despite the fact—of which the FDA was aware—that no scientific consensus existed on the safety of GM foods, even though some of the FDA's own scientists specifically questioned their safety. Thus, contrary to popular belief, the FDA does not formally approve GE crops as safe for human consumption; the GRAS review process of new, GE-food products involves only a voluntary consultation—one not nearly as rigorous as the testing of food additives—between the biotech companies and the agency.

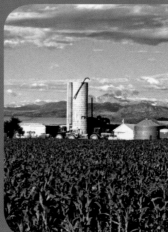

The biotech industry has played a key role in drafting the FDA policy on GE foods by lobbying, contributing to political campaigns, and perpetuating a dizzying revolving door among federal agencies and biotech companies such as Monsanto. And ultimately, the biotech industry got what it wanted: A tacit government endorsement of the safety of their novel foods and no regulation.

On March 21, 2000, the Center for Food Safety gathered an unprecedented coalition of scientific, consumer, environmental, and farm organizations. The group filed a legal petition with the FDA, demanding the development of a mandatory, thorough pre-market testing and labeling regime for GE foods. The group also called for the containment and reduction of existing GE crops. Members of the public can write in and support the action. You'll find more information on how to get involved at www.centerforfoodsafety.org.

FDA website on GE food: http://www.cfsan.fda.gov/~lrd/biotechm.htm

In 1977, scientists discover that the soil microbe, Agrobacterium tumefaciens, can transfer foreign genes to plants. Three years later, the U.S. Supreme Court sanctions the patenting of genetically engineered organisms, and by 1987, the first field tests of GE crops are underway on American soil.

The FDA's 1992 decision exempting genetically modified foods from federal regulation paves the way for a number of genetically engineered (GE) foods to enter U.S. markets.

The FDA approves Calgene's FlavrSavr tomato. The tomato flops with consumers because of its inferior flavor.

First U.S. planting of GE soy, followed by corn, potatoes, and cotton.

European Union declares a moratorium on the further development of GE products.

Kraft Foods recalls millions of dollars worth of taco shells after scientists discover StarLink corn, a GE crop that failed to meet EPA standards for human consumption, in their ingredients.

Monsanto Company pulls "New Leaf" GE potatoes from the market after McDonald's and Burger King pledge to serve GE-free french fries.

EU ends the moratorium on new GE products and institutes strict labeling and traceability requirements. The EU also establishes a rigorous approval process for future GE crops and foods.

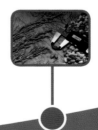

Brief History of Genetically Engineered Foods

For thousands of years, humans have changed the nature of their food, selecting, often unintentionally, desirable traits in the plants and animals they consume. Domestication and breeding are processes that alter an organism's genetic makeup to enhance its value to humans. Genetic engineering, however, departs from traditional techniques of plant modification by enabling the transfer of genetic material among unrelated organisms. A host of unknown risks to human health and the environment accompany this new technology.

1977   1992   1994   1996   1999   2000   2001   2004   TODAY

An estimated 87% of U.S. soy, 52% of U.S. corn, 55% of U.S. canola and 79% of U.S. cotton acreage are genetically engineered.[24]

ANTIBIOTIC RESISTANCE

As resistance genes spread across the world, powerful cures may start to fail. Every cell of many genetically engineered plants carries a gene that encodes resistance to antibiotics. When we eat these plants, antibiotic-resistance genes enter our bodies. Clearly, the biotech industry's irresponsible and widespread use of markers that carry genetic resistance to antibiotics (like ampicillin, a drug used widely in human medicine) could exacerbate the already-growing problem of antibiotic-resistant germs and reduce options for controlling infections. Spreading these resistance genes around the biosphere increases the chances of a dangerous germ picking up the gene and passing the immunity to other germs.

For almost ten years, the FDA has done worse than ignore its own scientists' warnings about antibiotic resistance: It has gone out of its way to dismiss their concerns in public. One official FDA statement concluded that "the likelihood of transfer of antibiotic resistance markers from plants to microorganisms in the gut or in the environment is remote and...would not add to existing levels of resistance in bacterial populations in any meaningful way."[25] But, contradicting its own contradiction, the FDA advised the pharmaceutical industry that if a genetically engineered food ingredient neutralized an antibiotic, "advice could be provided that the antibiotic should not be taken together with food."[26]

In other words, our food supply could undermine the use of powerful antibiotics. Yet instead of labeling the food, the FDA suggests marking the medicine bottle. Incidentally, the agency did not explain how patients should avoid consuming unidentified genetically modified foods. In May of 1998, just months before the FDA announced that antibiotic resistance markers were nothing to worry about, Patrice Courvalin, the chief antibiotics expert at the Louis Pasteur Institute in Paris, highlighted the potential for the transfer of resistance genes to bacteria in the digestive tract and in nature:

"We must remember that the opportunities for genetic exchange between living organisms in nature are immense...The intensive cultivation of plants carrying a resistance gene does result in the presence, in higher numbers, of this gene in nature, thereby creating the conditions that form its evolution and dissemination."[27]

While the FDA dithers and denies the risks of antibiotic resistance in genetically altered food, top health authorities and medical groups around the world face the danger head-on. The British Medical Association states:

"There should be a ban on the use of antibiotic resistance marker genes...as the risk to human health from antibiotic resistance developing in microorganisms is one of the major public health threats that will be faced in the twenty-first century."[28]

FACT

The FDA concluded that genetic engineering was a possible cause for the thirty-seven deaths and 1,500 disabling illnesses caused by the consumption of the dietary supplement L-tryptophan.

FACT

Our government continues to ignore the toxicity problem of GE foods. It has disregarded its own scientists, clear scientific evidence, and the possibility that genetic engineering can cause unintended changes in our food.

Toxic Genes

Some corporate scientists call genetic engineering a precise technology; the truth is it's anything but exact. Every time they insert a novel gene into a plant cell, the gene ends up in a random location in the plant's genome. As a result, each new gene amounts to a game of food-safety roulette, leaving companies hoping that the new gene, its cassette and whatever location it arrived in, will not destabilize a safe food and make it toxic.

The FDA has been well aware of this genetic-imprecision problem. Safety testing of the first GE food, the Calgene FlavrSavr tomato, uncovered stomach lesions in laboratory rats, and the agency knew it.[29] Even more significantly, the FDA concluded that genetic engineering was a possible cause for the thirty-seven deaths and 1,500 disabling illnesses caused by the consumption of the dietary supplement L-tryptophan.[30] Showa Denko, a Japanese company, used genetic engineering to produce the dietary supplement in the late 1980s. Apparently the engineering of this particular supplement may have created a toxic-contaminant byproduct that caused the deaths and illnesses.

Once again, our government was forewarned of the dangers presented by genetic engineering. Government scientists emphasized specifically that the genetic modification of these foods could result in increased levels of known, naturally occurring toxicants; the appearance of new, unidentified toxicants; and an increased capability of concentrating toxic substances from the environment (e.g., pesticides and heavy metals).[31]

Our government continues to ignore the toxicity problem of GE foods. It has disregarded its own scientists, clear scientific evidence, and the possibility that genetic engineering can cause unintended changes in our food that come with serious health consequences. To this day, mandatory FDA tests for the short- and long-term toxicity of GE foods don't exist.

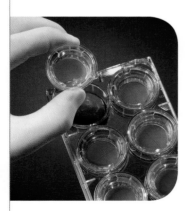
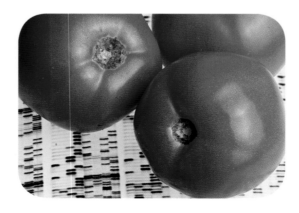
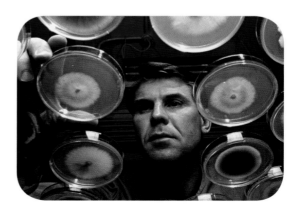

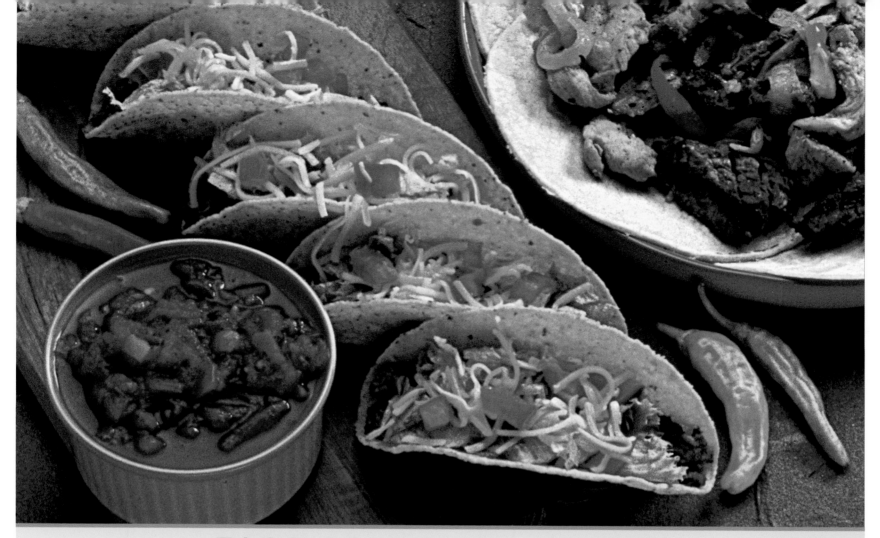

TACO BELL SHELL SHOCK

Think dangerous GE products can't enter the American food supply?

I n 2000, two public-interest groups arranged independent lab tests of Taco Bell® brand taco shells from Kraft Foods. The test found StarLink™, a genetically modified corn marketed by Aventis, in the shells.

The problem? Cattle could eat StarLink corn, but it was illegal for human consumption. Government experts warned that StarLink, modified to produce a pesticide protein called Cry9C, exhibited "characteristics of known allergens." Cry9C, like many allergens, is unchanged by cooking and can't be digested by humans.

Food safety groups demanded an immediate product recall. Under intense public pressure—in one of the biggest food recalls in history—more than 300 different products tainted with StarLink, and the pesticide protein Cry9C, were pulled off shelves across the country. Meanwhile, small amounts of StarLink continue to show up in our food. This episode begs larger questions: Why aren't food products adequately tested? What could be more important than protecting our food supply?

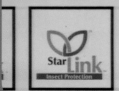

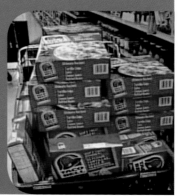

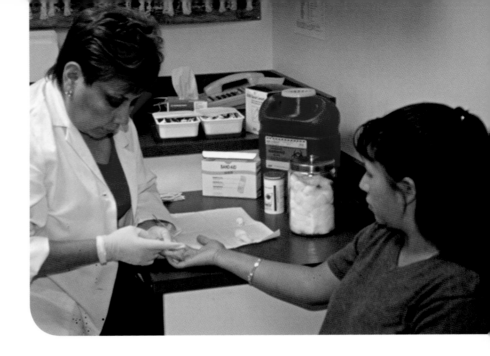

WEAKENING IMMUNE RESPONSE

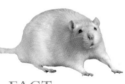

Besides the direct health perils of genetically modified foods, they may affect your body's ability to fight off other threats. In 1999, the respected United Kingdom journal, *The Lancet*, published a stunning report by Arpad Pusztai and Stanley W.B. Ewen and sponsored by the Scottish government.[32] The duo compared rats fed a regimen of genetically modified potatoes containing a natural pesticide called snowdrop lectin to rats that consumed potatoes without the lectin gene. Pusztai and Ewen found that rats on the genetically modified diet had underdeveloped organs, lower metabolism, and a less robust immune system.

Companies betting on genetic engineering have launched a campaign to discredit Pusztai and his research but have yet to present a single, peer-reviewed study refuting his observations. In fact, almost two dozen leading scientists have signed an open letter publicly defending the scholar and the validity of tests linking genetically modified foods to compromised immune response. And in May 2005, reports surfaced in the European press[33] that a secret 1,100-page study conducted by Monsanto on its GE corn, MON863, which is already grown and consumed in the U.S., found that rats fed a diet high in MON863 had significant differences in kidney weights and blood counts when compared with a control group. These results, considered "red flags" for possible impaired immune function and tumor growth, were seen to vindicate Pusztai and his research.

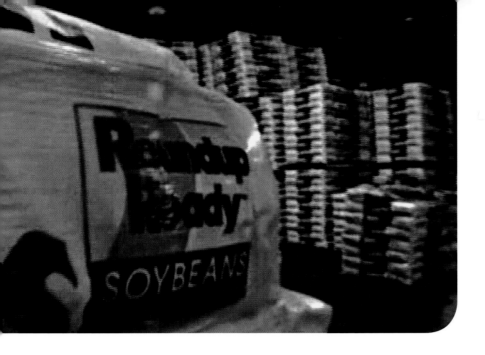

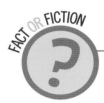

FACT OR FICTION

Genetic engineering is more effective than traditional plant breeding in producing desirable crops.

Fiction Genetic engineering has not proven to be more effective than traditional plant breeding. To cite just one example, traditional breeding was first to produce low-linolenic soybeans, which are used to create a healthier oil for use in processed foods.[37]

LOSS OF NUTRITION

The biotech industry often claims that someday it will come up with more nutritious food. Given the imprecision of the science and the massive failures it's experienced, these assertions are pretty much science fiction. One thing is for sure: Genetic engineering can lower the nutritional value of our current foods. In 1992, the FDA examined the problem of nutrient loss in GE foods. Their conclusion? Genetic engineering can result in "undesirable alteration in the level of nutrients" of foods.[34] The scientists also warned that these nutritional changes "might escape breeders' attention unless genetically engineered plants are evaluated specifically for these changes."[35] As of the publication date of this book, the government has not conducted such tests. In 1999, however, researchers at the California-based Center for Ethics and Toxics set out to do some testing of their own. Their results were published in a peer-reviewed scientific journal that same year.[36] They found that a common kind of genetically engineered soy, called Roundup Ready, showed a decline of 12 to 14 percent in types of plant-based estrogens called phytoestrogens. While the effects of phytoestrogens are debated, there is no question that these substances have important health effects given their ability to mimic human estrogens in the body. Phytoestrogens may offer protection against heart disease, osteoporosis (bone loss) and breast cancer. A 12-to-14-percent drop in these important elements is a significant nutritional difference. With soy products being present in a high percentage of our processed foods, this study indicates the urgent need of our government to begin the long-overdue task of determining the nutritional impacts of genetic engineering on our foods.

Who's who in agricultural biotechnology?

The technology of genetic engineering has changed little since its first commercial release in 1994. Four crops engineered to express two traits— herbicide tolerance (HT) and insect resistance (IR)—account for nearly every acre of commercial biotechnology. HT crops withstand direct spraying of weed killers while IR crops generate internal insecticides in their tissues. Among the four most common genetically altered crops, soybeans and canola are HT only; corn and cotton are HT and/or IR. Meanwhile, five biotechnology conglomerates dominate the market and contaminate our food supply:

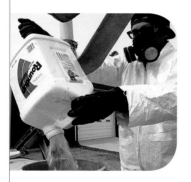

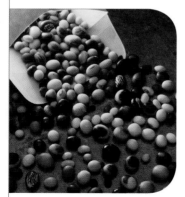

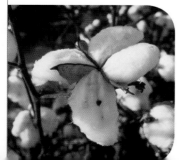

Monsanto Company: MONSANTO imagine·™

Monsanto Company is the world's undisputed plant-biotechnology leader. Ninety percent of the globe's genetically engineered crops harbor the company's seed traits.[38] Following the acquisition of Seminis, Inc. in early 2005, Monsanto became the world's largest seed company.[39] This biotech behemoth increased sales of its top-selling weed killer glyphosate—trade name Roundup—by linking its use to "Roundup Ready" HT seed varieties.[40] Monsanto's Roundup Ready versions of soybeans, corn, canola, and cotton are widely planted, and the company's Roundup Ready alfalfa recently hit the market with an uncertain future. Monsanto also manufactures the insect-resistant, "Yieldgard" corn. Despite this handful of commercial successes, many of Monsanto's approved biotech crops have failed in the marketplace. The long list of failed GE products includes Calgene's delayed-ripening tomatoes, insect-resistant tomatoes, Roundup Ready sugar beets, and insect- and virus-resistant potatoes.[41] Monsanto also produces the increasingly unpopular hormone rbGH, a hormone used in milk production and increasingly rejected by major dairies.[42]

DuPont: DUPONT™

DuPont owns Pioneer Hi-Bred International, Inc., and until Monsanto bought Seminis, Inc., was the largest seed company in the world. Although DuPont/Pioneer has few of its own GE crops on the market, the company is best known for its herbicide-resistant cotton variety, two types of insect-resistant corn, a sterile-pollen corn line used for breeding purposes, and nutritionally altered soybeans.[43] Though approved in the late 1990s for food use, these fat-altered soybeans have been rejected by food processors and are grown on only a few thousand acres in Iowa, exclusively for industrial use.[44] For the most part, DuPont/Pioneer sells insect-resistant corn hybrids containing Monsanto's trait (YieldGard) through licensing arrangements with Monsanto.

Dow Chemical Company: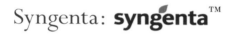

The Dow Chemical Company is the number one chemical manufacturer in the U.S. and second in the world.[45] Dow's agricultural biotechnology operations are run by two wholly owned subsidiaries: Dow AgroSciences and Mycogen Seeds, the latter acquired by Dow in 1998. Mycogen and Dow AgroSciences offer insect-resistant cotton, as well as two varieties of insect-resistant and herbicide-tolerant corn.[46] Mycogen sells other GM crop varieties under license from Monsanto. In September 2005, a longstanding patent dispute over the genetic engineering of insecticidal proteins into plants was resolved in Mycogen-Dow's favor. The patent decision gave Mycogen-Dow control over insecticidal traits from the soil bacterium Bacillus thuringiensis (Bt) in plants. Bt-based insecticides are used in all commercialized IR plants to date.

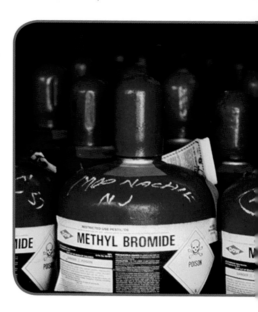

Syngenta: **syngenta**™

Syngenta formed when Novartis Seeds, the company's agricultural division, merged with Astra-Zeneca International's agribusiness operations in 2000. Not only does Syngenta rank among the world's top seed producers, the company is the globe's most prolific manufacturer of pesticides.[47] Syngenta makes atrazine, the nation's best-selling weed killer. The European Union banned the chemical because of its negative endocrine-disrupting effects.[48] Meanwhile, Syngenta's chief biotech product, Bt11, is an IR-field corn variety used mainly for animal feed and industrial uses. Interestingly, Bt11 sweet corn processed for human consumption is unpopular among farmers because of its universal rejection by food companies, such as the Del Monte Corporation. Syngenta, like the other agriculture biotech giants, has obtained licenses to incorporate Monsanto's traits into its own hybrids.

Bayer CropScience: Bayer CropScience™

United States environmentalists discovered that StarLink, a variety of GE corn unapproved for human consumption, had illegally contaminated the food supply, and hundreds of food products were recalled from supermarkets shelves across the country. The costs of compensating farmers, grain buyers, food companies, and consumers for the StarLink recall and its losses nearly topped $1 billion. The debacle ripened StarLink's developer, Aventis CropScience, for takeover by Bayer in 2002. Bayer CropScience is the world's second-largest seller of pesticides. Its CropScience division has inherited Aventis's biotech crops, which consist mainly of herbicide-tolerant versions of canola, cotton, and corn called "LibertyLink." Aventis's LibertyLink sugar beets, soy, and rice have been marketplace failures.

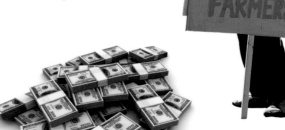

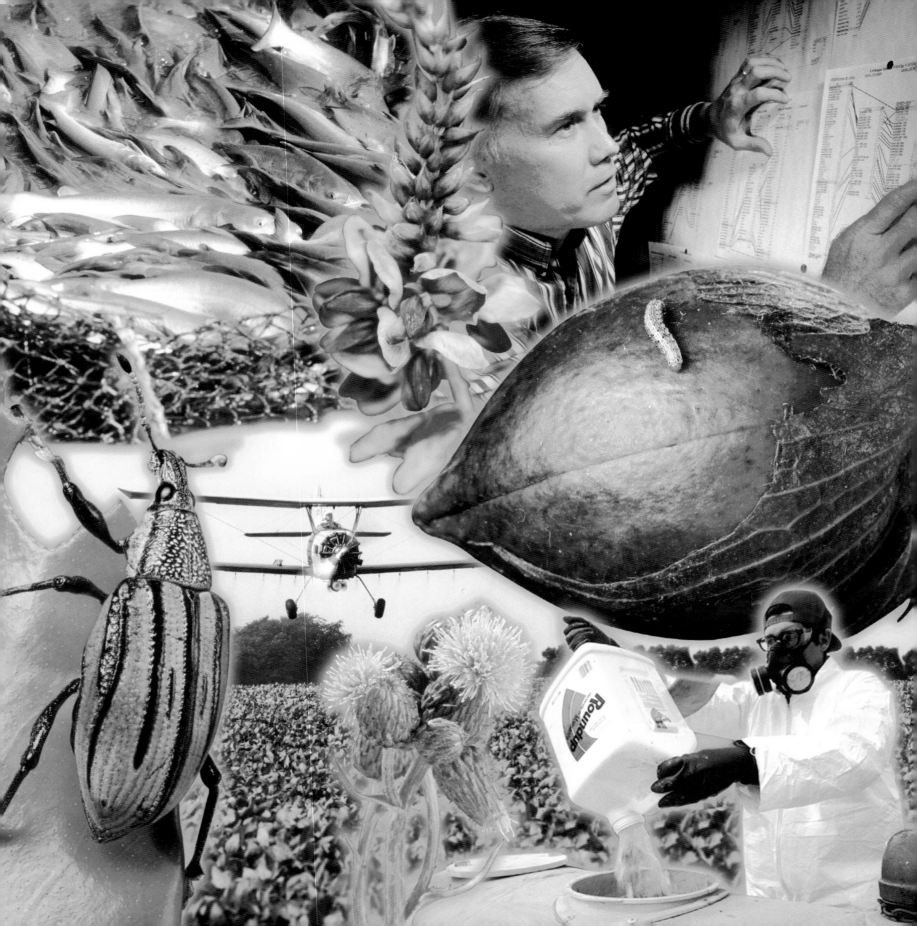

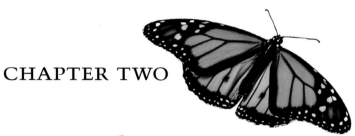

CHAPTER TWO

Ending Nature As We Know It

a Scientist speaks out

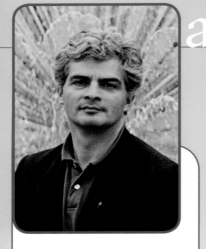

IGNACIO CHAPELA is a microbial ecologist and mycologist at the University of California, Berkeley, and an outspoken critic of the University's ties to the biotechnology industry. Chapela was finally awarded tenure in May 2005, after years of struggling against the undue influence of industry on the tenure-review process. Dr. Chapela is also the founder of the Mycological Facility, which investigates questions of natural resources and indigenous rights and is based in and run by indigenous communities in Oaxaca, Mexico.

IGNACIO CHAPELA, PH.D., ASSOCIATE PROFESSOR IN THE DIVISION OF ECOSYSTEM SCIENCES, UNIVERSITY OF CALIFORNIA, BERKELEY TELLS WHY HE'S CONCERNED ABOUT GE FOODS.

Q. Do you have any concerns about the process of genetic engineering plants?

The driving principles of how we do genetic engineering are extremely rudimentary— they don't take into account the most basic complexity that is necessary for the production of life. So we really do not have at this time, nor will we have in the foreseeable future, the capacity to reliably and reproducibly come up with any technological manipulation of life through DNA.

Q. Do you have any concerns about the genes being manipulated in genetically engineered (GE) organisms?

Yes. My concerns stem from something very fundamental in this manipulation of life. My concern has to do with the actual behavior of the pieces of DNA being "engineered" into these plants, not just of the plant that carries them. These pieces of DNA are unique. They themselves are made of mixed-and-matched pieces of DNA from other organisms that do very specific things. They are really promiscuous, that is, they insert themselves in any genome they find around. They also make themselves "very loud," meaning that they carry with them promoters that make them express themselves much more than any other gene would do in the unaltered plant. They carry all kinds of other functionalities—for example, antibiotic resistance or herbicide resistance—and you don't know what role those are going to play in the genome of the host organism. So, for me, the source of concern is this movement of DNA to foreign genomes where it shouldn't be. It is appropriate to envision this practice as the forced movement of a "DNA species" into a foreign "DNA ecosystem." Through painful and expensive experience, we know how serious the introduction of a biological species into the wrong ecosystem can be, and we should expect to see a similar effect with these manipulations at the molecular level.

Q. Do you think "co-existence" of GE and non-GE crops is possible?

No. It is not possible. I think this is a really important distinction: "co-existence" may be a convenient thing to have politically or commercially, but biologically, it is an impossibility. We know we are going to have transgene movement from a plant to other plants or weedy relatives over considerable distances—we just have to wait long enough. For most GMOs, the problem of contamination arises immediately; within one generation you have escaping genes. For others, such as self-pollinating or autogomous plants (e.g., soya and rice), it might take a little longer, but it will still occur.

Q: Why do you think it is important that GE crops do not spread in the environment?

There are so many reasons. First, the movement of transgenes and the organisms that carry those transgenes into the environment tend to reduce diversity and intensify the problems we already have with industrialized agriculture. So, for example, if agribusiness uses natural selection to create crops that are tolerant of herbicides, biotechnology uses genetic engineering to create plants with even more tolerance. With genetic engineering, a bad effect of industrial agriculture, the use of more herbicides, becomes multiplied.

Also, depending on which transgene escapes and where, you start worrying about a number of gene-pollution issues: species disruption or even extinction, the emergence of herbicide-resistant weeds, and effects on organisms that are not intended to be targeted.

Q. What do you think about companies being responsible for the safety testing of GE organisms?

It just confounds common sense to have companies being their own regulators. That cannot work because it is clearly not in their corporate interest to use sound science to find problems with their products. Even if they look hard enough to find a problem, history teaches us that they are far more likely to hide it than call attention to it.

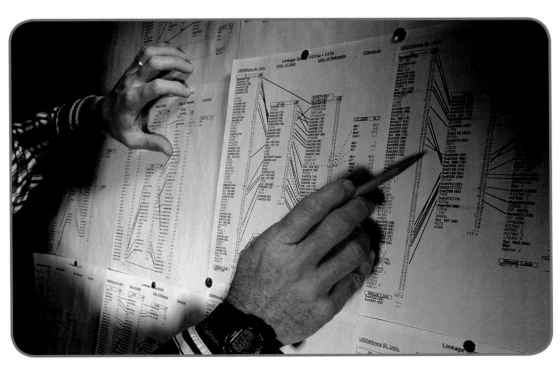

A Deal with the Devil

In November 1998, the University of California at Berkeley signed a controversial agreement with Novartis, one of the largest producers of GE seeds. Under this agreement, Novartis donated $25 million over five years to the University's Department of Plant and Microbial Biology. In exchange for these funds, Berkeley granted Novartis the first right to negotiate licenses on approximately one-third of scientific research conducted in the department, including discoveries funded with state and federal grants. The University also gave the company two out of five seats on the department's research committee which determined how the money would be spent. This deal caused tremendous dissent both within the student body and the university faculty and drew widespread media attention. As a result, in 2002 the university finally created an external research team to evaluate the controversial collaboration. The 2004 review findings concluded that the Berkeley-Novartis partnership "was outside the mainstream for research contracts with industry," and, they noted, "while an intriguing experiment, there appears to be little rationale for repeating the approach." In the meantime, such controversial public-private collaborations continue to flourish at public universities across the country.

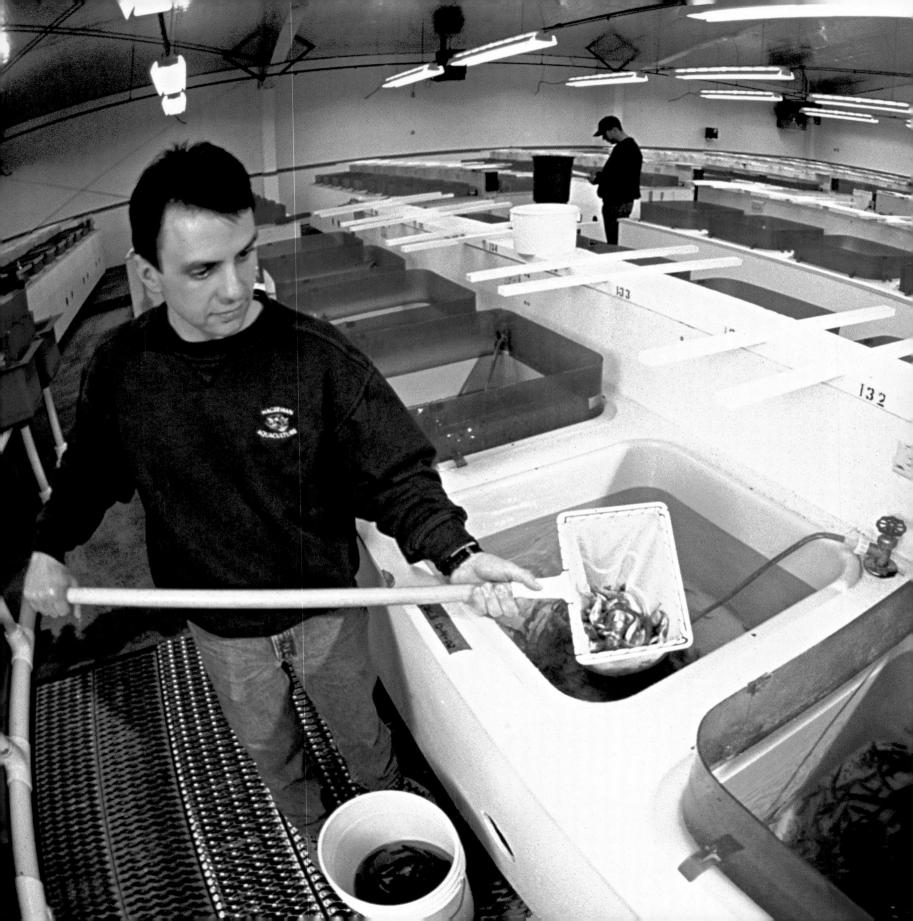

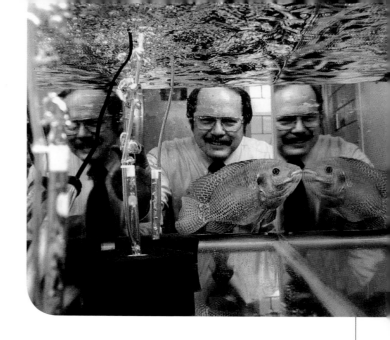

THE TROJAN GENE EFFECT

IT SOUNDS LIKE A SCIENCE-FICTION SCENARIO: engineer a fish with a gene for growth hormones to accelerate maturation and create a giant "super fish." Freakish as it may seem, for more than a decade, corporations and researchers in the U.S. and abroad have engineered human and other foreign growth genes into salmon, trout, and numerous other fish species in an attempt to make "super fish." Their incentive, of course, is to create a more profitable fish by taking a commercially viable fish, genetically engineering it to grow bigger faster, thereby bringing more seafood to the market in less time.

Lured by lucrative corporate profits, the research and development of genetically engineered seafood has increased in recent years. As of 2005, corporations and researchers worldwide are cobbling together at least thirty-five varieties of transgenic fish—fauna containing genes from foreign organisms.[1] Thanks to the legal and grassroots efforts of environmental and consumer groups, gene-altered seafood remains out of our supermarkets. But one company, Massachusetts-based Aqua Bounty Farms, continuously pressures the U.S. Food and Drug Administration to allow its engineered salmon, which can grow up to seven times faster than normal, in meat cases around the nation.[2]

FACT

Researchers found that if sixty genetically engineered fish joined a wild population of 60,000 fish, this population would vanish within forty generations.

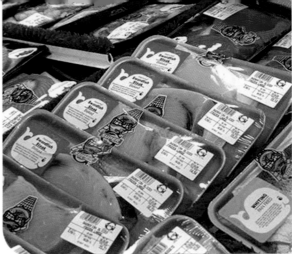

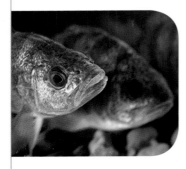

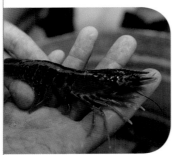

While corporations continue to engineer fish and push for their commercial use, scientific evidence mounts regarding the extraordinary environmental dangers these fish pose. Several recent studies suggest that the release of these fish into open waters could be catastrophic. In 1999, a study by William Muir and Richard Howard of Purdue University revealed that these super fish could wipe out local, wild populations of a species.[4]

Muir and Howard discovered that fast-growing genetically engineered fish have a reproductive advantage over wild fish. It turns out that fish prefer super fish when mating. But there's a catch. Because of the unnatural growth genes passed down to them, the offspring of these fish have a high and early mortality rate: genetically engineered fish are three times more likely to die prematurely than wild fish. The growth gene that gives super fish the reproductive advantage spreads through the native population quickly, and soon, native fish populations could dwindle and eventually become extinct.

"You have the very strange situation where the least-fit individual in the population [the genetically modified fish] is getting all the matings—this is the reverse of Darwin's model," said Professor Muir. "Sexual selection drives the gene into the population and the reduced viability drives the population to extinction."[5] The researchers found that if sixty genetically engineered fish joined a wild population of 60,000 fish, this population would vanish within forty generations. Subsequent research has shown that extinction could occur even quicker. Even one transgenic fish could have the same devastating impact, though extinction would take longer.

The two Purdue researchers have dubbed this extinction scenario the Trojan Gene Effect. "This resembles the Trojan Horse," according to Professor Muir. "It [the growth gene] gets into the population looking like something good and it ends up destroying the population."[6]

As corporations and researchers multiply the numbers of these super fish, there is increasing concern that the destructive potential of the Trojan Gene Effect will be realized. Wild salmon are exceptionally vulnerable to this blight. Even the release of a few of the genetically engineered salmon pending commercial approval could obliterate Atlantic salmon, a species already threatened. A genetically altered salmon, intentionally or accidentally introduced into the wild, could not be recalled, found, and destroyed. Instead, it would survive, mate, and contaminate a native population with its growth gene. The 114 varieties of endangered fish, including populations of Chinook, Coho, and Sockeye salmon, are especially at risk from the proliferation of transgenic fish. Should a Trojan gene make its way into any one of these vulnerable populations, extinction could result.

And extinction is forever.

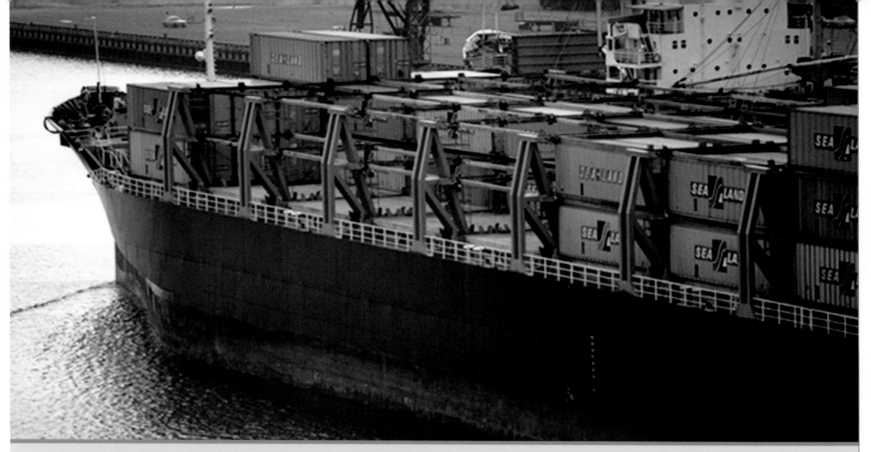

INTERNATIONAL REGULATION OF GMOS

The rest of the world has been leaps and bounds ahead of the U.S. when it comes to regulating GE foods.

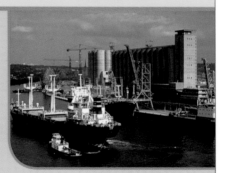

The Cartagena BioSafety Protocol, effective September 2003, is the first piece of international legislation that regulates the trans-border trade of genetically engineered organisms. More than 140 countries have ratified the protocol, allowing them to ban the import of genetically modified products deemed a threat to human and animal health and the environment. The protocol also stipulates that genetically modified products slated for export must be appropriately labeled.

Only a handful of countries, including the U.S., Canada, Argentina, Australia, Chile, and Uruguay, currently export GMOs. With the exception of the United States and Australia, all have since signed the agreement. The U.S. continues to dispute GE food bans sanctioned by the Cartagena Protocol, citing violations of free-trade agreements. Supporters of the legislation maintain that "free trade" is not truly free without the consumers' informed consent.

Nearly sixty countries require the labeling of genetically modified foods, or in some way restrict its growth and import. Russia, Saudi Arabia, China, Mexico, Brazil, and South Africa are among the countries that have adopted labeling requirements. Additionally, regional governments in countries worldwide have created GE-free zones by banning cultivation of GE crops at the local level.

In May 2004, the European Commission lifted a five-year de facto moratorium on GE products. However, all GE foods imported to the EU must still be approved by the European Commission. The EU also requires the labeling and traceability of all GE foods and ingredients.

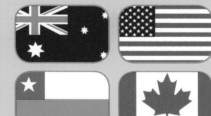

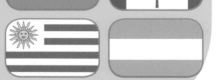

Cartagena Protocol website: http://www.biodiv.org/biosafety/

Some experimental GE fish and shellfish*

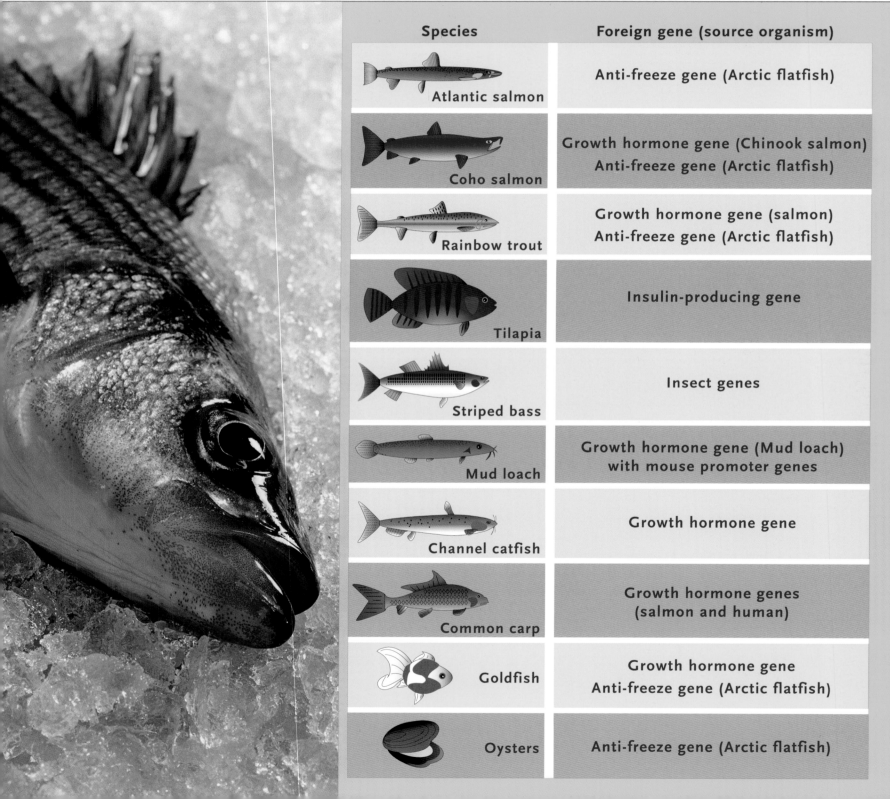

Species	Foreign gene (source organism)
Atlantic salmon	Anti-freeze gene (Arctic flatfish)
Coho salmon	Growth hormone gene (Chinook salmon) Anti-freeze gene (Arctic flatfish)
Rainbow trout	Growth hormone gene (salmon) Anti-freeze gene (Arctic flatfish)
Tilapia	Insulin-producing gene
Striped bass	Insect genes
Mud loach	Growth hormone gene (Mud loach) with mouse promoter genes
Channel catfish	Growth hormone gene
Common carp	Growth hormone genes (salmon and human)
Goldfish	Growth hormone gene Anti-freeze gene (Arctic flatfish)
Oysters	Anti-freeze gene (Arctic flatfish)

*Source: Adapted from the FAO's report, The State of the World Fisheries and Aquaculture 2000, p.73, ftp://ftp.fao.org/docrep/fao/003/x8002e/x8002e00.pdf

Desired effect(s)	Country
Cold tolerance	U.S. Canada
After 1 year, 10- to 30-fold growth increase	Canada
Increased growth and feed efficiency	U.S. Canada
Production of human insulin for diabetics	Canada
Disease resistance, still in early stages of research	U.S.
Increased growth and feed efficiency; 2- to 30-fold increase in growth; inheritable transgene	China Rep. of Korea
33% growth improvement in culture conditions	U.S.
150% growth improvement in culture conditions; improved disease resistance; tolerance of low oxygen level	U.S. China
Increased growth	China
Increased growth	U.S.

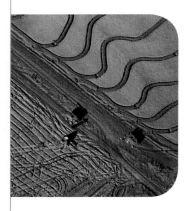
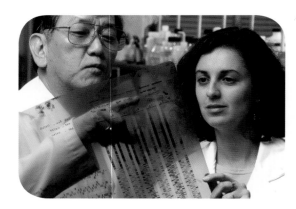
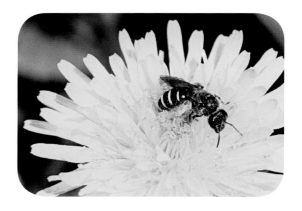

BIOLOGICAL POLLUTION

RICE CRISIS ‹

In early 2006, an unapproved, genetically engineered rice known as LL601 was found to have contaminated commercial long-grain rice supplies throughout the U.S. The illegal rice had never undergone USDA review for potential environmental impacts required prior to marketing, nor review by the FDA for possible harm to human health. As a result, Japan immediately suspended imports of U.S. long-grain rice, and rice prices fell dramatically.

This episode is just one of many incidents of an illegal GE crop contaminating the food supply, and shows the USDA's continuing failure to adequately regulate and monitor field testing of GE crops. The Center for Food Safety has called upon the USDA to enact a moratorium on all new permits for open-air field testing of GE crops until the agency demonstrates it can keep these unapproved varieties out of the food supply.

We all know about the chemical pollution that contaminates our air, water, and soil. But we don't think much about the living organisms—viruses like the bird flu, the fungi that causes Dutch elm and chestnut blight diseases, plants like the kudzu vine, and animals such as zebra mussels or killer bees—which can engender so much havoc on humans and the environment. Like these naturally occurring biological pollutants, genetically engineered life forms born in the test tube can quickly knock nature irreversibly off balance.

Gene-altered fish and the stockpile of genetically modified corn, soy, and cotton plants grown in the U.S. are also exotic, meaning they have not evolved in the ecosystem into which they are introduced. In fact, these organic anomalies have never existed anywhere outside a Petri dish. Yet these organisms are released into the environment with little or no assessment of the risks they represent. Unlike chemical pollutants, which ooze into the environment over time, biological pollutants reproduce, disseminate, and mutate. They do not degrade as chemicals do and cannot be cleaned up like a chemical spill. Instead, biological pollutants multiply exponentially; control and recall efforts are futile.

The DNA from genetically engineered plants does escape and cause harm, according to a 2004 report by the National Research Council of the National Academy of Sciences.[8] The report suggested that the control of further gene propagation and the environmental harm that could accompany it will be difficult, if not impossible, to constrain. The report urged the "stringent bioconfinement" of many crops to keep genetically modified organisms from escaping into the wild gene pool. The study also concluded that no method was 100 percent effective. Underscoring the insurmountable task of controlling living pollution, a 2004 study authored by an EPA scientist demonstrated that genetically engineered grass could contaminate native flora more than thirteen miles away.[9] Nevertheless, biotech companies continue to gush out their biological pollutants over millions of acres despite the findings and the warnings issued by independent scientists.

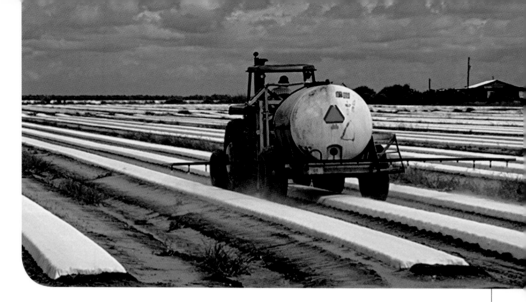

HERBICIDE HEAVEN

Currently, four out of every five acres of genetically engineered crops in the United States and around the world are engineered to be herbicide-tolerant (HT).[11] Foreign genes help these crops tolerate ever-increasing amounts of herbicide application. To facilitate herbicide use by farmers and to expand the market for weed killers, Monsanto and other chemical companies created herbicide-tolerant crops. These altered crops also addressed a major problem that chemical manufacturers faced when weeds became resistant to years of treatment with their top-selling herbicides such as Monsanto's Roundup.[12] As a result, farmers had to spray more and more herbicide on their crops to kill these weeds. But herbicides kill crops too, compounding the weed issue for increasing numbers of farmers. These designer plants were concocted to withstand ever-growing doses of herbicide. In this sense, Monsanto engaged in a kind of planned obsolescence. Roundup Ready crops facilitate massive increases in herbicide use, resulting in a higher resistance to weeds. In the long run, Roundup Ready treatments

would be ineffective; in the short term, the added weed resistance meant a spike in the sales and profits of Roundup and resistant seeds. The scheme worked. Greater sales of chemicals and herbicide-tolerant seeds, like Monsanto's Roundup Ready products, have translated into hefty profits for Monsanto and other biotech conglomerates.

Monsanto's gain is nature's tragedy and our loss—HT crops require exponential increases of certain herbicides to remain effective. Data from the biotech industry reveal that herbicide use has grown substantially because of these gene-altered plants,[13] a fact that government data corroborate. One researcher using federal figures estimated an increase of more than 138 million pounds of herbicide to treat U.S. fields since 1996.[14] This means ever-more chemical pollution of our fields, waters, air, and food and the devastation of the diversity of organisms on agricultural lands. A recent three-year study revealed that ongoing herbicide use on these resistant crops could decrease wildlife including bee, butterfly, and bird populations by 30 percent.[15]

Genetically engineered crops can decrease the amount of wildlife in farm fields.

Fact A U.K. study found that fields of genetically engineered, herbicide-tolerant canola and beets hosted fewer bees and butterflies than conventional fields. This result was likely due to changes in weed vegetation caused by the herbicide use program for the GE crops.[10]

"The genetically engineered crops now being grown represent a massive uncontrolled experiment whose outcome is inherently unpredictable. The results could be catastrophic."[7]

—*Barry Commoner, Ph.D.*
Senior Scientist at the Center for Biology of Natural Systems at Queen's College, City University of New York

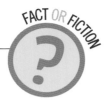

Roundup is a relatively harmless herbicide.

Fiction In an experiment mimicking the conditions of an aquatic ecosystem, a University of Pittsburgh researcher found that Roundup was lethal to amphibians. "Roundup reduced tadpole [species] richness by 70 percent by completely exterminating two species (leopard frogs and gray tree frogs) and nearly exterminated a third species (wood frogs)."[16]

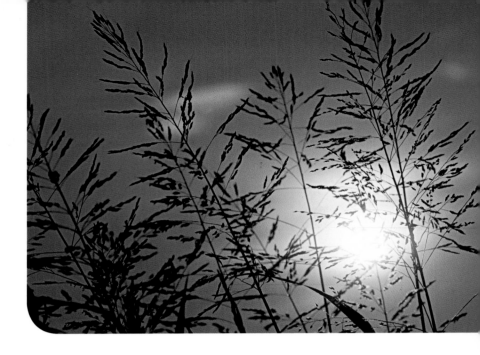

THE DAWN OF THE "SUPER WEEDS"

FACT
Roundup-resistant horseweed now infests over a million acres across about a dozen states.

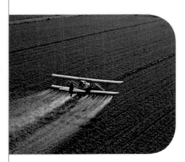

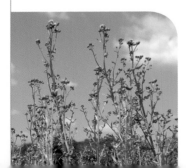

Engineering a plant to tolerate ever-greater amounts of a chemical herbicide not only encourages the use of more chemical pollutants, but also increases the serious problem of herbicide-resistant weeds. Therefore, as these herbicide-resistant super weeds become harder and harder to eradicate, they will require even larger amounts of lethal chemicals, in turn delivering more dangerous pollution to the environment. The first herbicide-resistant weed, horseweed, was found in a GE crop in 2001.[17] The contamination of horseweed occurred where Roundup Ready soybeans were grown for several years without rotating crops. The Roundup-resistant horseweed now infests over a million acres across about a dozen states.[18] Since that time, other Roundup-resistant weeds have developed, forcing the use of even more toxic herbicides.[19]

Even scientists at Calgene, the company that introduced the first commercial genetically modified crop, noted in 1985: "The sexual transfer of genes to weedy species to create a more persistent weed is probably the greatest environmental risk of planting a new variety of crop species."[20]

Genetically engineered crops can also become super weeds themselves. In the late 1990s, canola farmers in Alberta, Canada began planting three kinds of seeds designed to withstand commercial herbicides. One was genetically modified to resist Monsanto's Roundup, another stood up to Aventis LP's Liberty herbicide, and the other seed was tolerant of Cyanamid's Pursuit and Odyssey weed killers. By early 2000, farmers were surprised to find canola plants

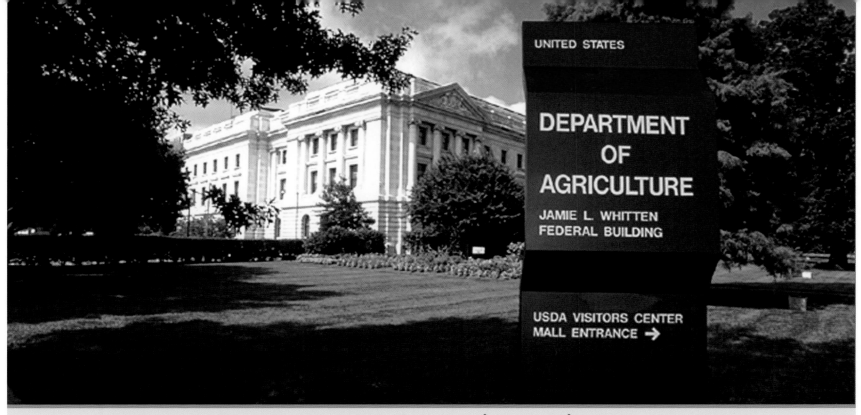

YOUR TAX DOLLARS (NOT) AT WORK

EPA and USDA Asleep on the Job.

The three agencies that share most of the responsibility for regulating genetically engineered crops are the Food and Drug Administration (FDA), the Environmental Protection Agency (EPA), and the U.S. Department of Agriculture (USDA). The EPA and USDA are responsible for regulating the environmental impacts of GE crops.

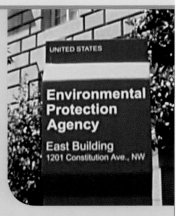

The EPA oversees crops containing internal pesticides; the agency only regulates the pesticide, not the plant. For instance, the EPA has jurisdiction over the *Bt* pesticide in *Bt* corn, but the FDA governs the corn itself. Plants engineered with a trait such as herbicide tolerance elude EPA environmental review. Meanwhile, the EPA has failed to delve into the long-term risks associated with GE crops, ever-more common throughout the U.S.

The USDA regulates genetically engineered foods through one of its divisions, the Animal and Plant Health Inspection Service (APHIS). USDA's oversight includes the interstate movement and importation of plant-pest organisms, as well as the field-testing of GE crops.

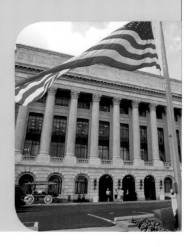

The USDA decides consistently to deregulate crops submitted for environmental review by biotech companies. Deregulation allows the sale and cultivation of the crop by exempting the parent crop and its progeny from the USDA's regulatory authority. In 2002, a committee of the National Academy of Sciences reviewed the USDA's crop-supervision performance.[21] The committee found a lack of transparency, too little external scientific and public review of the agency's decision-making, and poorly trained personnel.

As a result, new GE crops are being rubber-stamped by federal agencies despite evidence that proves these crops will contaminate native and conventional plants and pose other significant new environmental threats.

USDA website on GE crops: www.aphis.usda.gov/brs/

EPA website on GE crops: www.epa.gov/pesticides/biopesticides

Experimental GE field trials in the U.S.: www.nbiap.vt.edu/cfdocs/fieldtests1.cfm

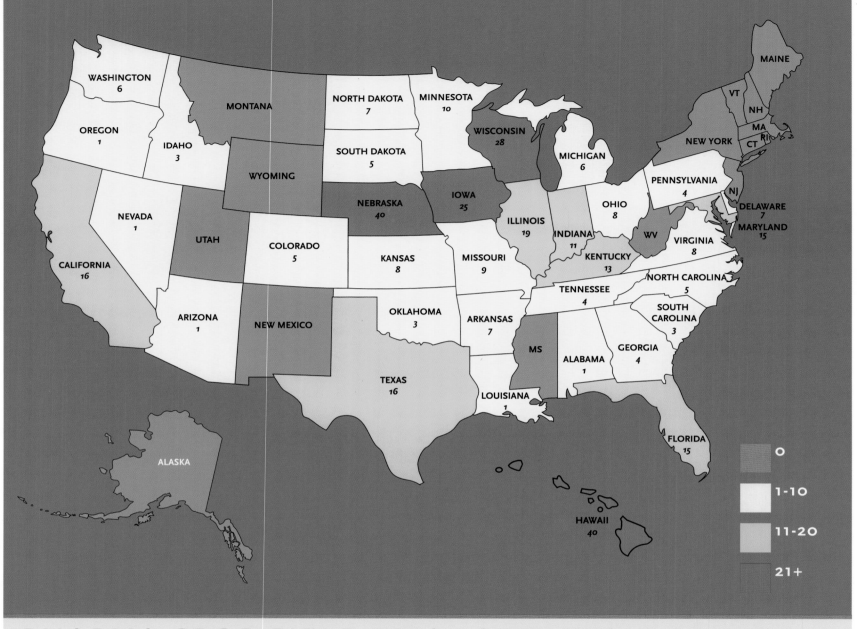

WASHINGTON 6

OREGON 1

IDAHO 3

MONTANA

NORTH DAKOTA 7

MINNESOTA 10

WISCONSIN 28

MICHIGAN 6

MAINE

VT

NH

MA

NEW YORK

RI

CT

NEVADA 1

WYOMING

SOUTH DAKOTA 5

IOWA 25

ILLINOIS 19

INDIANA 11

OHIO 8

PENNSYLVANIA 4

NJ

DELAWARE 7

MARYLAND 15

CALIFORNIA 16

UTAH

COLORADO 5

NEBRASKA 40

KANSAS 8

MISSOURI 9

WV

KENTUCKY 13

VIRGINIA 8

NORTH CAROLINA 5

ARIZONA 1

NEW MEXICO

OKLAHOMA 3

ARKANSAS 7

TENNESSEE 4

SOUTH CAROLINA 3

TEXAS 16

MS

ALABAMA 1

GEORGIA 4

LOUISIANA 1

FLORIDA 15

ALASKA

HAWAII 40

Legend:
- 0
- 1-10
- 11-20
- 21+

PHARMA CROP FIELD TRIAL APPROVALS PER STATE

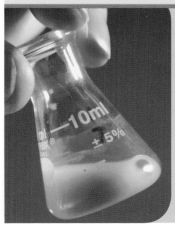

Union of Concerned Scientists

"**P**harma crops" are plants that have been genetically engineered to produce pharmaceutical or industrial chemicals. Currently, no drugs from such plants are on the market. But pharma crops are being tested in our collective backyard. Common food crops such as corn or rice are often used—raising the specter of drugs contaminating our food supply. This map shows the estimated number of USDA-approved plantings of pharma crops in each state, from 1991 to 2004. To learn more, visit the Union of Concerned Scientists at www.ucsusa.org.

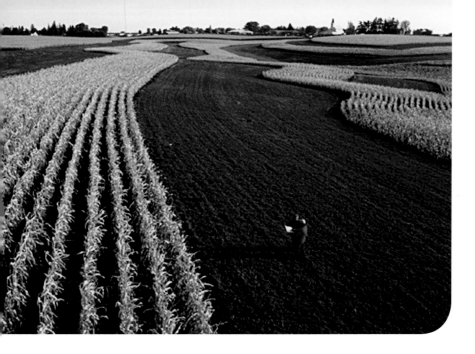

growing in and around their fields that resisted all three herbicides.[22]

This was bad news for Canadian wheat, bean, and barley farmers. As triple-resistant canola spreads across Alberta, farmers' options for controlling these super herbicide-resistant "volunteer" canola plants will diminish, necessitating the use of the most toxic herbicides for eradication. In the words of the Royal Society of Canada, "volunteer canola could become one of Canada's most serious weed problems."[23]

Some biotech advocates claim buffer zones will shield wild-weed varieties from genetically modified crops, thereby easing the bio-pollution threat of super weeds. But buffer zones would offer at best an imperfect solution, and as mentioned earlier, crops with long pollen flow distances render the idea of buffer zones impractical. Moreover, a 2003 British study[24] found that some cross-pollination among genetically modified plants and their weedy relatives, regardless of the distance between species, was inevitable.

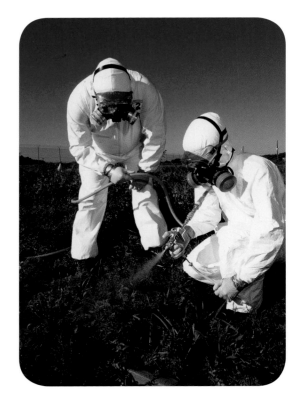

FACT

Engineering a plant to tolerate ever-greater amounts of a chemical herbicide not only encourages the use of more chemical pollutants, but also increases the serious problem of herbicide-resistant weeds.

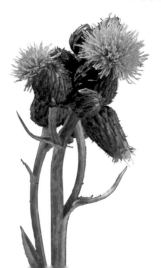

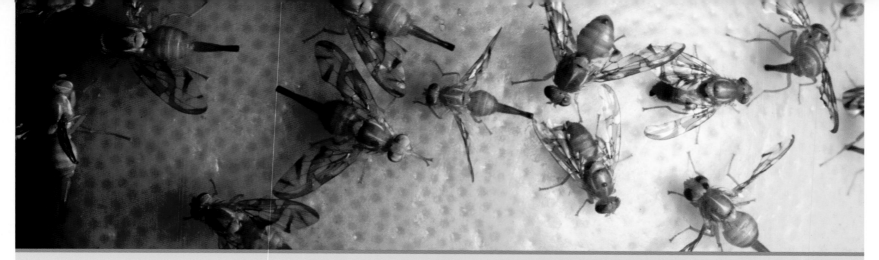

FALSE PROMISES

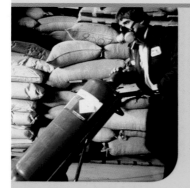

GE crops were supposed to lead to less pesticide use. But have they?

The biotech industry promises that their inventions will make the world less dependent on agricultural chemicals. But crops genetically modified to tolerate farm poisons and to resist diseases and pest insects generate their own biological pollution. Research shows that, over the long term, genetic modification will boost the use of chemicals rather than reduce it. In recent years, U.S. Department of Agriculture data show that with widespread planting of genetically modified crops, pesticide reliance has actually grown. According to a recent study, in the past nine years, 122 million more pounds of pesticides have been applied to farm fields due to the introduction of genetically modified crops.[26] Why?

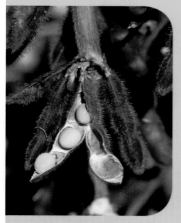

Widely grown herbicide-resistant crops necessitate the increase of pesticide treatments. A biotech industry—funded study found that herbicide use is commensurate with the number of herbicide-resistant crops.[27] During the first three years of the widespread harvesting of Roundup Ready soy, the industry's study determined a 14 percent overall gain in herbicide application; per-acre use also increased significantly.[28] Soybean growers who plant Roundup-resistant crops are employing more and more Roundup and other chemicals to manipulate crops in their favor.[29] A plant modified to tolerate a chemical herbicide obviously encourages the grower to use more of that particular herbicide. And when an herbicide-resistant weed multiplies as a result of this practice, it will persist and spread among farmers' fields.

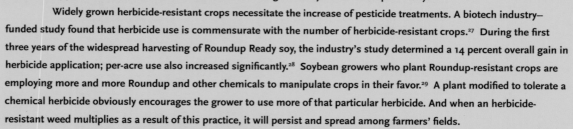

What about *Bt* crops? Will they reduce the use of harmful insecticides? While some data indicate that *Bt* crops have so far reduced the reliance on non-*Bt* insecticides, the long-term picture is by no means promising. While genetically engineered *Bt* plants eliminate some pests, other bugs find new opportunities, and to curb their crop destruction, require larger amounts of pesticides. For example, some North Carolina farmers who grew the first generation of cotton *Bt* crops found that these crops failed to deliver a pest-control panacea. Although the *Bt* did eliminate some bugs, it also created new infestation opportunities, which had never been a major threat to cotton before. These southern farmers suddenly saw stink-bugs swarming around their *Bt* fields.[30] The growers retaliated by spraying large amounts of organophosphate insecticides. A 1999 study predicted this problem. It stated that when a potato modified to resist the Colorado potato beetle succeeded in controlling the beetle, it opened up a biological niche for aphids.[31] The aphids, unharmed by the potato's modified genes, and in the absence of the chemical insecticides that previously controlled them, devoured the crop.

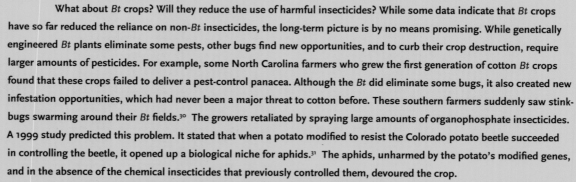

Just as modifying plants to tolerate weed killers sucks conventional growers even deeper into chemical agriculture, genetic modifications pumping out more *Bt* toxins will accelerate *Bt* resistance—driving some organic farmers out of business or back to harmful chemical pesticides.

In short, the GE crop–filled future looks bleaker, not brighter.

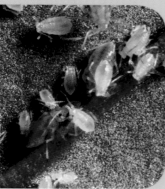

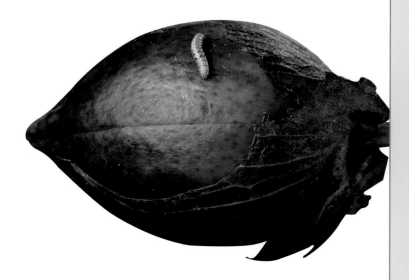

EVERY FIELD A PESTICIDE FACTORY

As plants are programmed to tolerate weed killers, so are they modified to produce their own pesticides. One naturally occurring bacteria—Bacillus thuringiensis (*Bt*)—generates proteins that are toxic to various pests. Sprayed on crops and then exposed to sunlight, *Bt* breaks down quickly and poses few risks.[32] And because it's a natural pesticide, *Bt* is especially important to organic farmers who are permitted to use non-synthetic pesticides.

But turning food crops into pesticide-producing plants is different from an occasional spraying. As one scientist explains of a *Bt* cotton, "This practice amounts to a continuous spraying of an entire plant with the toxin, except the application is from inside out."[33] As a result, genetically modified plants create *Bt* toxins at high levels and over long periods of time, as compared to plants sprayed by farmers only when needed.[34] The toxin is even emitted from the roots of some *Bt* crops, creating a subterranean pesticide-zone with unknown consequences for the biological community in the soil.[35]

Above ground, the effects of *Bt* crops are troubling too. In a controlled experiment, pollen from genetically modified corn was dusted on the leaves of milkweed plants. *Bt* toxin in the corn pollen boosted the death rate of monarch butterfly larvae that fed on the milkweed.[36] Could the same thing happen in real life? Researchers found that the concentration of *Bt* in the pollen of one variety, *Bt*176, was sufficient to kill monarchs on milkweed in and near cornfields in northern states where monarch larvae are present when corn is producing pollen.[37] In a related study, *Bt*176 interfered with the normal development of harmless black swallowtail butterflies.[38] Eventually, Syngenta was forced to take *Bt*176 off the market.[39] Luckily, *Bt*176 was never widely grown—deterred neither by the altruism of regulatory agencies nor the conscience of biotech companies, but by the constraints of economics.

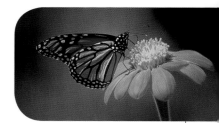

FACT

The threat to monarch and black swallowtail butterflies was narrowly averted when *Bt*176 was withdrawn from the market.

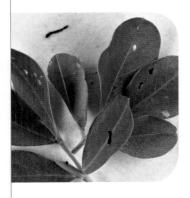
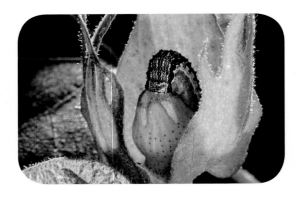
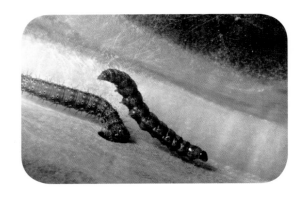

BREEDING SUPER PESTS

Ironically, turning crops into pesticide producers may simply speed the day when pests develop resistance to *Bt*, just as they do to artificial insecticides. We know it's possible. Researchers watched diamond-back moths become fully tolerant after just two dozen generations—about eight crop seasons—of feeding on *Bt* broccoli.[41] Field studies on commercial crops have not been conclusive, but many researchers and farmers consider *Bt* resistance a serious threat. The farmers' fears were substantiated in 2005 when a *Bt*-resistant strain of cotton bollworm was identified in Australia.[42] If *Bt* tolerance spreads, this low-impact pesticide will become useless. Biotech's exploitation of *Bt* is leading to a new generation of pests the bacteria can't touch. The biggest losers will be consumers, organic farmers, and conventional farmers who use microbial *Bt* to reduce our exposure to more toxic insecticides. Nearly half of organic growers say they spray *Bt* regularly or occasionally.[43] Without *Bt*, they would have to choose between crop losses and pricier control techniques. Both could increase consumer prices for organic foods and cut demand.

The biotech companies' misuse of *Bt* represents a serious and lasting threat to the survival of organic farming in the United States. As *Bt* is compromised, many organic farmers will have to abandon their certifications and sustainable practices and return to chemical pesticides. Others may stop farming entirely. If chemical-intensive agriculture muscles out organic farming, consumers will experience a significant reduction in the supply of organic food and a tragic end to farming alternatives.

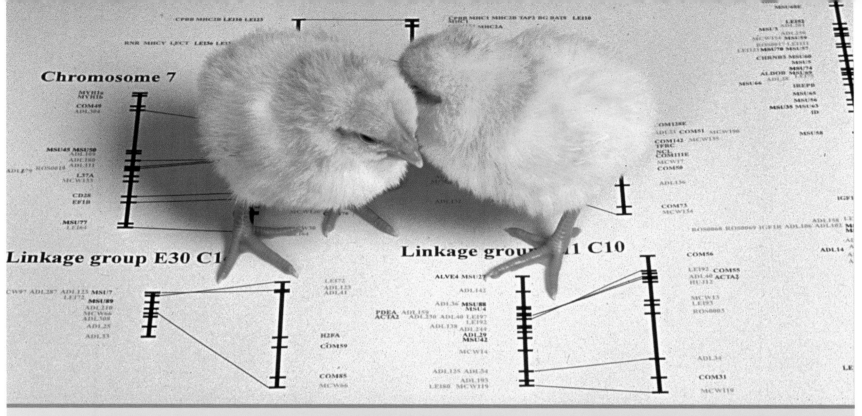

GENETICALLY ENGINEERED AND CLONED ANIMALS

Animal Welfare Concerns

Animal welfare issues abound with rbGH, and the same is true of new animal technologies. Biotechnology companies are developing cloned and genetically engineered (GE) breeds of virtually every animal species used for food. The industry is currently awaiting FDA approval to market GE fish and milk from cloned dairy cows, and genetic engineers are developing cloned and/or GE varieties for pork, beef, eggs and poultry, and lamb production.

In animal cloning, unsuccessful reproduction is by far the norm; in many animals, cloning fails to produce healthy offspring 95 to 97 percent of the time.[44] Severe pregnancy complications in cloned cows are common, as are defects such as grossly oversized calves, enlarged tongues, squashed faces, intestinal blockages, immune deficiencies, and diabetes.[45] Problems in other cloned animals include these as well as high rates of heart and lung damage, kidney failure, and brain abnormalities.[46]

Cloning may inherently cause health problems in animals. In 1999, scientists writing in *The Lancet* reported the first evidence that cloning may have long-term harmful effects that are not apparent at birth or even weeks later. The researchers concluded that factors inherent to the cloning process or faulty regulation of genetic development during somatic reprogramming caused the death of their cloned cow.[47] Genetic engineering includes these and other potential animal welfare concerns. (While genetic engineering and cloning are distinct technologies, they are often used in tandem.) The National Academy of Sciences has warned that "unexpected phenotypic effects, especially on anatomical, physiological, or behavioral traits of genetically engineered animals can occur."[48] In fact, such unanticipated effects are common in transgenic animals. For example, Canada's leading scientific society stated that the potential for side effects associated with genetic engineering is "the rule rather than the exception in fish."[49] As the industry moves to bring food from cloned and transgenic animals to market, needless animal suffering will be dramatically increased.

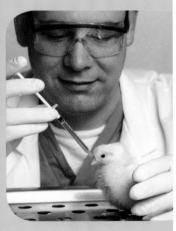

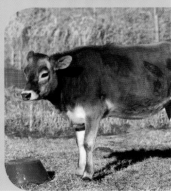

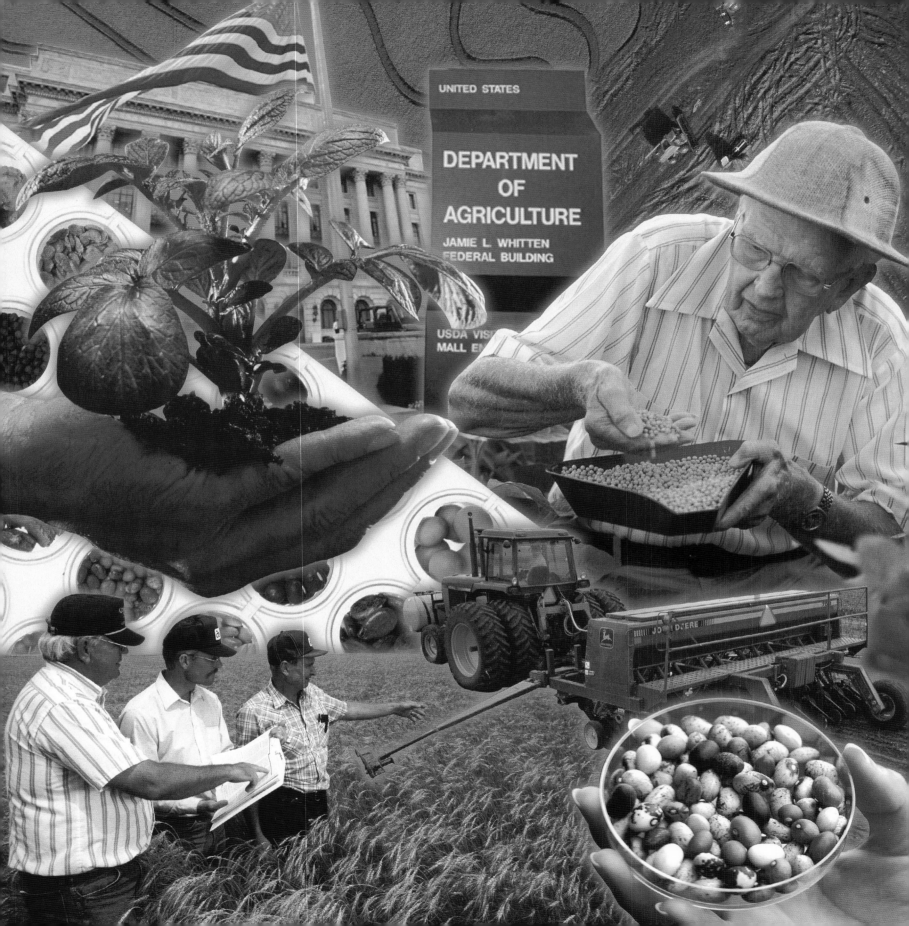

UNITED STATES

DEPARTMENT
OF
AGRICULTURE

JAMIE L. WHITTEN
FEDERAL BUILDING

USDA VIS
MALL EN

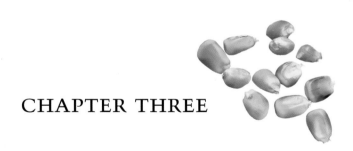

CHAPTER THREE

Sowing Seeds of Destruction

a Farmer speaks out

Marc Loiselle, organic farmer in Saskatchewan, Canada, tells why he's concerned about GE foods.

Marc Loiselle was born in the far northern Saskatchewan community of Île-à-la-Crosse. Today he manages an organic farm in Saskatchewan, where he grows wheat, barley, oats, and rye and raises goats and chickens. Loiselle has led a crusade to protect Canadian farmers against the potential economic losses related to the cultivation of GM crops. This includes filing an organic farmers' class action lawsuit against Monsanto for financial losses due to widespread contamination of Canadian canola.

I am an organic farmer. The motto of our organic farming organization is "Food For Life." We take this vision seriously and we mean "LIFE" in its most positive senses. We mean that the food we produce must be life-giving and must promote health and longevity. We also mean that the system we use to produce that food must not be a threat to ourselves, other humans, or other species. We organic producers, in the process of making our livings, must treat the land and its flora and fauna with the utmost respect. The Food for Life system needs to be economically viable, environmentally sound, and socially just, while also meeting the needs of today and not compromising the needs of future generations.

The organic farming techniques we use have fed humankind for thousands of years. Organic farmers reject the philosophy that we must poison our environment and use the radical genetic engineering of plants and animals to produce enough food for everyone to eat. In fact, genetic engineering leads to less yield, not more. Moreover, organic certification standards and the Food for Life ethic absolutely prohibit the use of genetically modified organisms. The organic market depends on farmers being able to supply food that is produced without toxic and damaging input, including GMOs. If we cannot guarantee a product free of contamination, we are not able to service those markets, resulting in a loss of our ability to be financially sustainable and a loss of choice for you, the consumer.

As organic producers, we are, of course, directly affected by the introduction of GMOs. GE varieties such as canola, corn, and soybeans cannot be contained within specific research plots or farmers' fields because their novel traits drift from field to field. Pollen and seed disbursements caused by wind, water, and animal and human activity spread these traits. Without guarantees that we can grow and market non-GMO contaminated crops, we risk losing our certifications and our livelihoods.

If, as a farmer, you use GE material, you are contributing to this biological pollution of our crops. You are also exacerbating the international corporate control of our seeds and of our food and ensuring the disenfranchisement of your fellow farmers. If growers don't take a united stand for limits on biotechnology and on seed patenting, we risk losing market access, income, choice, and control over what we produce, how we produce it, its value, and who will buy it.

We farmers are deeply disturbed by how transnational companies have promoted genetic engineering and obscured its risks to human health and the environment. What's more, these corporations keep GE foods unlabeled, manipulate legislatures into exempting them from liability, and do not disclose their own studies.

Biotech conglomerates and their friends in government want the food system to conform to their designs. In their quest for the uniformity of food production, these entities have totally ignored the dangers to biodiversity and the rights of farmers and consumers. Unfortunately, many governments continue to support biotechnology with increasing fervor. We believe that if a significant portion of the money used to foster agricultural biotechnology were shifted to the backing of farmers, sustainable agriculture, and the safety of the public and the environment, humanity would be much better served.

Meanwhile, the biotechnology industry asks us farmers to trust them. But how can we trust them when these companies persecute farmers, preclude us from decisions that affect our futures, and pressure us into giving up control of our land and seeds? How are we to ever believe that any good will come of biotechnology for food development, given its track record over the years? Shame on our governments, institutions, and public agencies for allowing the corporate takeover of our agricultural resources. The only reason all of this engineering of food and seed patenting is happening in the first place is the old story of money and greed.

In sum, the bio-engineered agribusiness approach to food production is completely incompatible with the Food for Life vision. It threatens to reduce farmers to serfdom, perpetuates the use of toxins and genetic engineering in food production, and offers little or no diversity of choice for consumers. Some say that the development of GE crops and foods has gone so far that the only thing left to do is to accept it, lick our wounds, and try to get compensated for our losses. We say that's unacceptable—and dead wrong. It's not too late to halt the genetic engineering and patenting of our seeds, but we'll all have to join together to stop it.

For more information about the Saskatchewan Organic Directorate, visit www.saskorganic.com

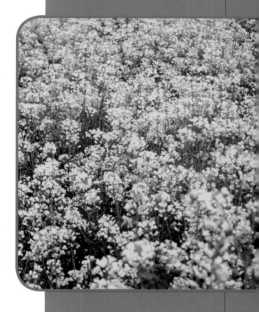

"Organic farmers reject the philosophy that we must poison our environment and use the radical genetic engineering of plants and animals to produce enough food for everyone to eat. In fact, genetic engineering leads to less yield, not more."

My Manifesto

I am a passionate supporter of organic farming.

I am a steward of an intergenerational family farm.

I believe in farmers' rights to grow and save their own seeds.

I believe all people have the fundamental right to unpolluted air, water, soil, and food.

I believe governments need to empower people—and need to redirect their policies towards truly sustainable agriculture.

I believe consumers are the ultimate market, that they know best what to eat, and that they have the right to choose.

I believe in the common good.

I believe that no life forms should be patented—including seeds—and that there must be agreement on sharing the genetic commons. It is a collective responsibility, not to be claimed as intellectual property.

I don't believe in using poison or genetic engineering to produce food.

I don't believe in the eventual domination of the food industry by a few transnational companies.

I don't believe in farmers being married to grain, chemical, or GE companies.

I care about the environment and people's health and welfare.

I care about what we eat and how we grow it.

I care about having neighbors and vibrant rural communities.

I want people to care about the way I grow food.

I want justice for all farmers and consumers.

I want the freedom to remain a farmer and to be able to grow what I want without GMOs.

I want my children to have the freedom to farm.

I want everyone to have abundant life.

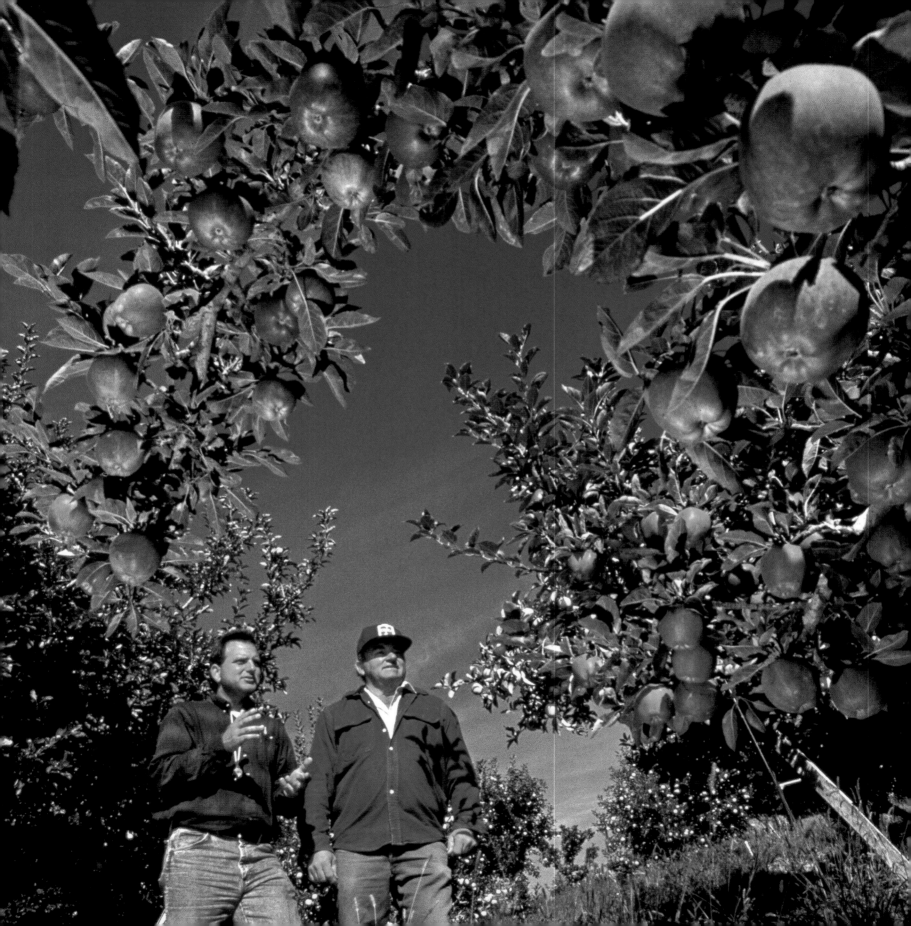

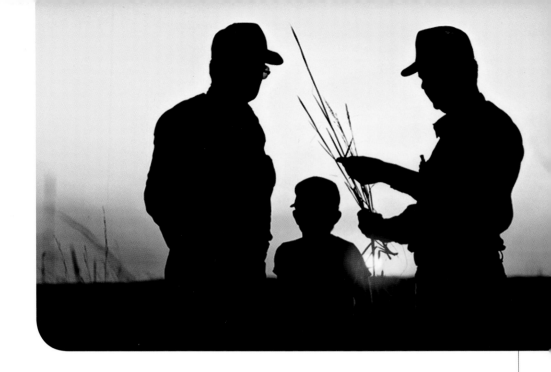

WHERE HAVE ALL THE FARMERS GONE?

OVER THE LAST HALF-CENTURY, as chemical-intensive farming has come to dominate U.S. agriculture, the number of farms and farmers has been drastically reduced, rural communities have been decimated, and profits have been concentrated among large corporations.

Despite agribusiness promises that new technologies will lead to safer, more successful farms, farming has become one of the most dangerous, most stressful, least stable, and least profitable professions in the United States. While food retailers and chemical, biotechnology, and seed companies grow richer and more powerful, increasing numbers of farmers are forced to abandon their farms and file for bankruptcy. Their suicide rate is also one of the highest of any profession in the country.[1]

Farmers in the U.S. and abroad are told that adopting genetic engineering is the answer to their problems. But today, almost ten years after biotech conglomerates commercialized genetically modified crops in North America, many farmers are realizing that biotechnology is a large part of the problem instead of a solution. Take the experience of Tom and Gail Wiley, family farmers in North Dakota.

"The lethal use of genetic engineering biotechnology threatens the food security of this and future generations. It destroys the very basis of the livelihood systems which our ancestors have developed for centuries, finely adapting to the diverse ecosystems in which they have evolved."[2]

—*Professor Wangari Maathai*
Founder of the Kenyan Green Belt Movement, 2004 Nobel Peace Prize Winner

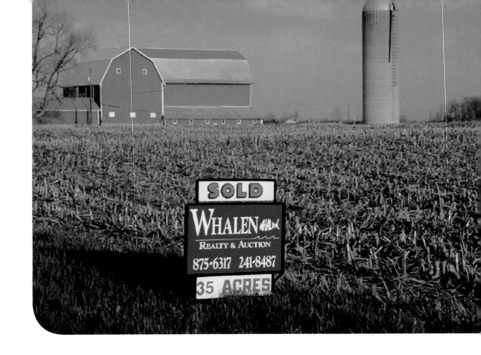

LOSING MARKETS, LOSING FARMS

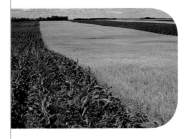

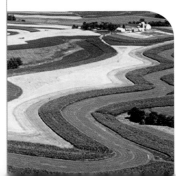

The Wileys' farm produces about 1,000 acres of soybeans every year. When offered genetically modified seeds, they refused. "I have not seen any reason to go the GE route," Tom said. The Wileys did not know it at that time, but their choice to avoid GE crops would not matter. In 2000, soon after eschewing the GE option, Tom landed a lucrative contract to grow food-grade soy for Japan—an opportunity that would safeguard their livelihood. Just as they were about to deliver their soy, the Wileys received shocking news. Their prospective buyers tested the crop and found a major problem: the soy contained a 1.37-percent GE contamination. Because Japan prohibits GE soy, the contract was canceled. The Wileys were left empty-handed, wondering how their farm got contaminated.[3]

The Wileys are not alone. The United Kingdom's Soil Association chronicled the grim economic reality of GMOs: U.S. farmers have already lost more than $300 million in annual corn export sales to Europe because of tainted crops and the possibility of GMO contamination.[4] These losses contribute to an estimated $3 to 5 billion-a-year drain on the U.S. economy, from lower farm prices and associated increases in U.S. crop subsidies.[5] Now, because the European Union (EU) requires the labeling and traceability of genetically modified ingredients, the U.S. State Department expects export losses to dramatically increase.[6]

Clearly, the biological pollution caused by genetically engineered pollen and seed is becoming a monumental financial problem for the farmers of today and the

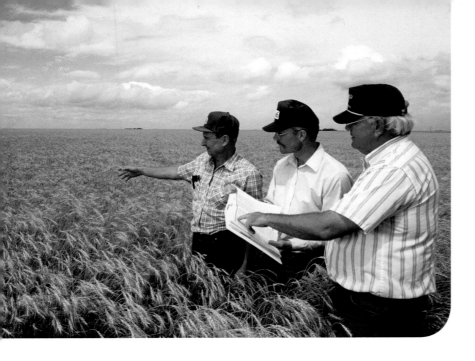

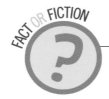

GE crops threaten the future of organic farming.

Fact GE crops threaten organic farming in two ways. First, the widespread use of *Bt* crops is likely to hasten insect resistance to microbial *Bt*, thereby undermining an important natural insect repellant used by organic farmers. Second, contamination of organic fields with GE traits threatens the market for organic products, which consumers expect to be produced without the use of GE.

future. Containing the GM plague is impossible, because wind, rain, birds, and other vectors can indiscriminately carry seeds. A 2003 U.K. study found that genetically modified canola, our main source of vegetable oil, can cross-pollinate with conventional canola located more than sixteen miles away.[7] The same study discovered that insects carry pollen six times farther than earlier studies anticipated. Another U.K. study[8] disclosed the immediate and long-term damage of crop defilement: GE canola can contaminate conventional and organic varieties for more than sixteen years. A scientist with our own Environmental Protection Agency discovered that one GE grass can spread its genes over a large surrounding area, pollinating related plants more than thirteen miles away.[9] While the biotechnology companies reap profits on altered agricultural products,

farmers like the Wileys ultimately pay the price.

Genetically altered material can also sneak into seed stocks, making uncontaminated seed ever-more difficult to find. A recent Union of Concerned Scientists report revealed that genetically modified varieties contaminate 50 to 80 percent of conventional corn and soybeans and 80 to 100 percent of traditional canola seed stock.[10] In some areas, conventional seed companies and organic farmers have stopped growing certain crops because they can't produce a field free of genetically modified material. This pollution of seeds increases risks to conventional farmers and seriously jeopardizes the future of organic agriculture.

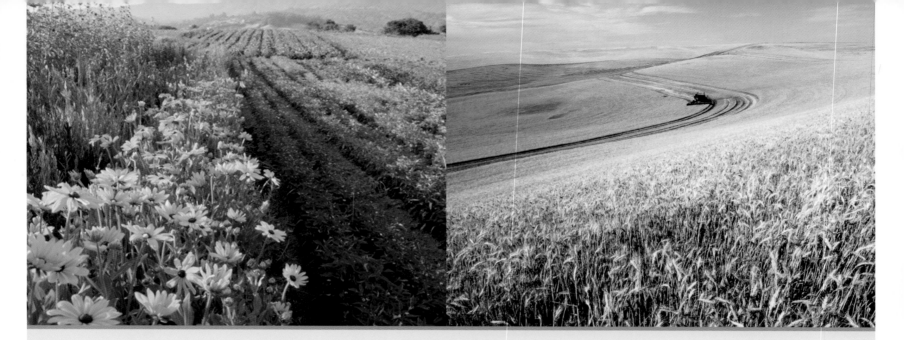

ROBUST DIVERSITY OR
FRAGILE MONOCULTURE?

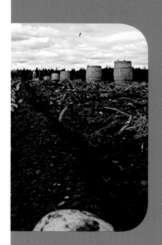

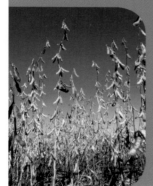

From the beginning, the biotech industry has claimed that genetic engineering will make agriculture more environmentally sound. However, a robust environment depends on diversity, whereas industrial agriculture aims for just the opposite: uniformity. "Monocultures"—enormous expanses of farmland planted with a single variety of a single crop—are designed for mechanization and chemical control. With the rise of these farming practices has come a decrease in diversity. For example, while more than 5,000 varieties of potatoes are grown worldwide,[11] Russet potatoes, the kind used in McDonald's french fries, account for 70 percent of the U.S. crop.[12] The U.N. Food and Agriculture Organization estimates that three-fourths of agricultural genetic diversity has been lost in the past century.[13] Genetically modifying crops doesn't solve the problem of so-called monocropping—it makes it worse.

Instead, biotech companies are sinking ever greater amounts of research dollars into developing new, patentable, genetically modified varieties, causing sales of conventional seeds to decline as the biotech seed sector grows.[14] Unusual seed varieties are omitted from commercial catalogs[15] and made unavailable to growers and seed breeders, giving way to biotech domination.

Even high-quality conventional seeds are hard to find. "You can't even purchase them in this market. They're not available," says soybean farmer Troy Roush of Van Buren, Indiana. A cotton farmer from Texas reports, "Just about the only cottonseed you can get these days is Bollgard or Roundup Ready. Same thing with the corn varieties. There are not too many seeds available that are not genetically altered in some way."

Meanwhile, penalties for seed saving discourage farmers from breeding varieties most suitable to their climate, soil and pest conditions. Whereas ten thousand years of settled agriculture discovered 50,000 kinds of edible plants,[16] a mere fifteen crops provide 90 percent of the world's food energy intake today.[17] Among those crops, varieties have shrunk to a small handful controlled by corporate patents.

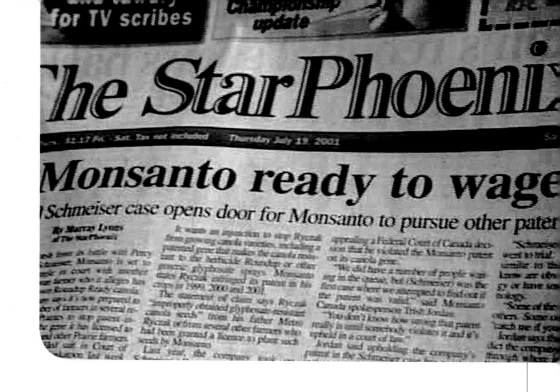

GENETIC ENGINEERING AND THE PERSECUTION OF FARMERS

Bio-pollution is just one consequence of genetic engineering that threatens the American farmer. The danger of seed patents is another. Biotechnology companies, especially Monsanto, have stifled the millennia-old agricultural practice of saving, exchanging, and sharing crop seeds. They have deterred farmers from saving and trading their seeds by obtaining patents, a practice our government has allowed for the last twenty years. (For a discussion of what this has done to agricultural biodiversity, see left, "Robust Diversity or Fragile Monoculture?")

Monsanto and other biotech companies have taken full advantage of this unfortunate policy decision, thereby acquiring a multitude of patents on both genetic engineering techniques and genetically engineered seeds. Their patent domination is abetted by an important fact: plants reproduce and, in the process, can spread their genes to other plants. Patented genes will follow the reproductive stream as far as a pollen grain or new seed will travel. When patented traits contaminate non-genetically engineered agriculture, the tainted crop effectively becomes the property of these companies. And like the Wileys, farmers who unknowingly sow patented technology can then be prosecuted for violating seed patents.

Consider the case of Percy Schmeiser.[18] The seventy-four-year-old farmer works his

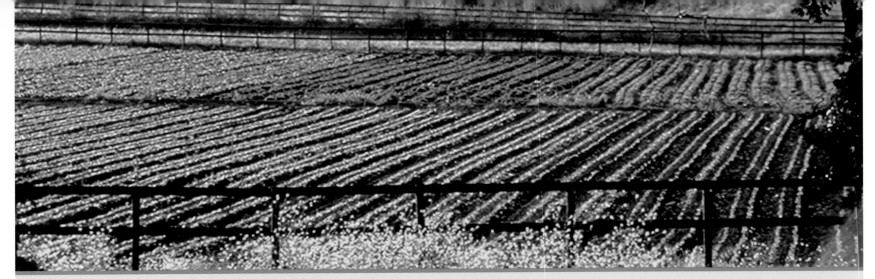

HOW GE THREATENS THE SURVIVAL OF ORGANIC

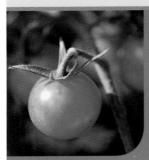

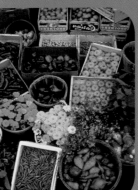

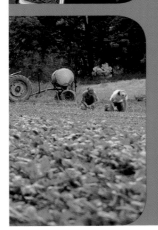

Organic agriculture has emerged as the fastest-growing sector in American agriculture, year after year. However even as the organic movement continuously rises in popularity and profitability, genetic engineering threatens to sabotage this vital new movement. GE and the companies that promote it present two potentially lethal threats to organic agriculture:

1) Contamination undermines the right of organic farmers not to grow GE.

Consumers rightly expect that organic foods are produced without the use of genetically engineered seed. But genetic engineering is uncontainable by its very nature. Organic crops and seeds have been contaminated with GE material via inadvertent seed mixing, pollen flow, and other means. And even though the presence of GE material alone does not necessarily constitute a violation of the organic regulations, the marketplace (e.g., consumers, marketers, and food processors) will often reject foods with any presence of GE material. As a result, organic farmers can and are suffering economic losses. Farmers and food processors are also incurring increased costs to test their products to be sure they are GE-free.

How to halt this assault on organic? First, stop the introduction of any new GE crops. Next, for those crops already planted, force the biotech companies that produce these altered seeds to have full liability for any added costs to organic farmers including the testing of their seeds, purchasing of non-contaminated seeds, and market losses due to contamination.

2) GE insecticidal plants could compromise an important tool for the organic farmer.

Aside from herbicide tolerance, the most common kind of genetic engineering involves taking a gene for an organic pesticide called *Bt*, and putting it into each cell of the crop. The idea is for the crop to create its own pesticide and kill the insects that prey on it. In its natural form in the bacteria Bacillus thuringiensis, *Bt* is a major tool that organic farmers have as a non-synthetic pest-deterrent. Used on a small scale and sprayed as needed, there is a low chance that insects will become resistant to *Bt*. But in GE crops the insecticide is typically produced all the time, in all parts of the plant, across very large fields. Such an environment is likely to foster *Bt* resistance in pests. Biotech companies are not worried; the end of *Bt*'s effectiveness would signal the opportunity for a new insecticide or insecticidal crop. But for organic farmers, some of whom rely on *Bt*, this resistance is disastrous as it deprives them of a valuable solution to the pest problem. It could even force some farmers back into the use of harmful, synthetic pesticides.

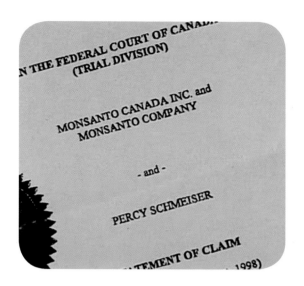 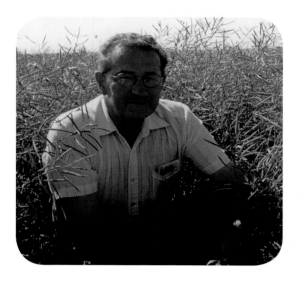 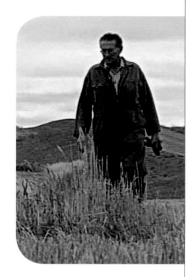

land outside Bruno, Saskatchewan. Monsanto sued Schmeiser in 1998, alleging that he'd planted and profited from its patented Roundup Ready canola seeds. The company demanded Schmeiser pay back the money he made from his crop.

Percy Schmeiser refused. He pointed out that he never bought any of the GE seeds and that he'd simply followed his usual practice of collecting seeds from his own crop to plant the following year. He claimed the contamination occurred from genetically modified canola grown nearby or Monsanto seed dropped on the roads bordering his fields. He argued that he was not responsible for the blight of his crop by Monsanto's product. Monsanto countered that regardless of how its patented crop showed up on Schmeiser's farm, the company was entitled to royalties. Remarkably, the lower courts in Canada agreed with Monsanto's position. But Schmeiser was undeterred. He appealed the case all the way to the Canadian Supreme Court. "I got thrown into something that I never ever wanted to be in," he says. "I'd rather be fishing with my grandkids. But now that I'm in it, I don't regret the deci-

sion. I don't want to be a hero or a saint. But, by God, there comes a time when you've got to take a stand."

In 2004, the Canadian high court handed down a mixed decision.[19] Unfortunately, they ruled that Monsanto's patent on herbicide-resistant canola seed was valid— but they also released Schmeiser from paying damages to Monsanto because the presence of patented GE material added no value to his crops.

Still, this judgment could seriously hamper Monsanto's ability to prosecute Canadian farmers for patent violations. If the company is only entitled to collect profits generated by its technology, Monsanto will not amass anything in these lawsuits. Not only does GE technology not add value to crops, it often makes them unmarketable. Schmeiser is considered a hero among small-scale farming communities and groups around the world opposed to the proliferation of genetically modified organisms. And the Schmeisers' fight continues: Percy's wife Louise recently sued Monsanto for contaminating her organic home garden.

FACT

U.S. farmers have already lost more than $300 million in annual corn export sales to Europe because of tainted crops and the possibility of GMO contamination.

"I am someone who fundamentally believes that patents are for toasters, not for living things."[20]

—*Winona LaDuke,*
Native American activist, environmentalist, economist and author

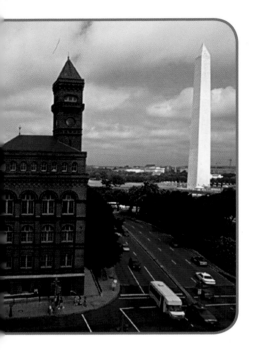

To ensure marketplace success and international acceptance, biotech companies have developed strategies to influence the United States government in their favor. The leaders of biotech companies not only foster important relationships with regulators and elected officials worldwide, but also possess key policymaking positions in Washington D.C. Thus, companies like Monsanto have dictated policy to many federal agencies, including the U.S. Department of Agriculture (USDA), the Environmental Protection Agency (EPA), and the Food and Drug Administration (FDA). It's all part of the Revolving Door, a term that refers to the movement from biotech company leader to government policymaker and vice versa. To understand just how prevalent the effects of the Revolving Door have been, let's take a look at the people who've been through it.[21]

MONSANTO COMPANY

LINDA FISHER, former EPA deputy and assistant administrator. Before joining the EPA, she spent five years as a Monsanto Company executive. Before that, she practiced law at Latham & Watkins, a firm known for fighting tougher regulatory standards on behalf of powerful industry clients. Fisher left the EPA in 2003 to become DuPont's Vice President and Chief Sustainability Officer.

MARGARET MILLER, past chemical laboratory supervisor for Monsanto who worked on the bovine growth hormone. She is now the FDA's Deputy Director of Human Food Safety and Consultative Services.

MICHAEL A. FRIEDMAN, MD, former acting Commissioner of the FDA Department of Health and Human Services, now Senior Vice President for Clinical Affairs at GD Searle & Co., a pharmaceutical division of the Monsanto Company.

MARCIA HALE, former President Bill Clinton's past assistant for intergovernmental relations, now Director of International Government Affairs for Monsanto Company.

MICHAEL (MICKEY) KANTOR, erstwhile U.S. Secretary of Commerce and former United States trade representative and then-member of the board of directors of Monsanto Company.

MICHAEL TAYLOR, former legal adviser to the FDA's Bureau of Medical Devices and Bureau of Foods, and Executive Assistant to the Commissioner of the FDA. Later, he was a partner at the Atlanta law firm

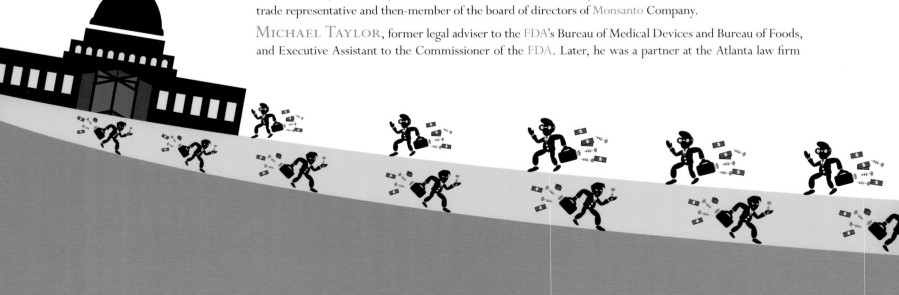

King & Spaulding where he supervised a nine-lawyer group whose clientele included Monsanto Company. Then he served as the FDA's Deputy Commissioner for Policy before returning to King & Spaulding. He later headed the Washington, D.C. office of Monsanto Company.

JOHN ASHCROFT, former U.S. Attorney General. Out of 535 members of the House of Representatives and the Senate, he received the greatest amount of financial support from Monsanto; he collected five times more money than the Congressman finishing second.

ANNE VENEMAN, former director of Calgene—absorbed by Monsanto and now part of Pharmacia Corp.— the biotech company that introduced the world's first genetically altered food, the FlavrSavr tomato. Later, she became the USDA's Secretary of Agriculture.

CLARENCE THOMAS, a Monsanto lawyer who became a United States Supreme Court Justice. He wrote the majority of the Supreme Court policies that allow the patenting of plants.

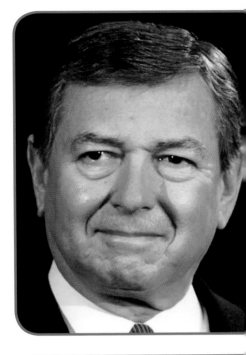

OTHER BIOTECH CONNECTIONS

L. VAL GIDDINGS, former senior staff geneticist, international team leader, and branch chief for science and policy coordination of the USDA's Animal and Plant Health Inspection Service (APHIS), biotechnology products regulatory division. Hired by the Biotechnology Industry Organization as Vice President of Food and Agriculture.

DAVID W. BEIER managed Genentech, Inc.'s government affairs; served as chief domestic policy adviser to Al Gore, former Vice President of the United States.

TERRY MEDLEY, former administrator of the USDA's Animal and Plant Health Inspection Service. Previous administrator of the FDA food advisory committee; currently Director of Global and Corporate Regulatory Affairs for DuPont

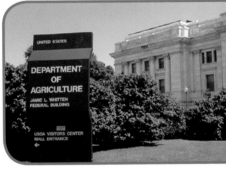

MICHAEL PHILLIPS, one-time director of the board on agriculture and natural resources for the National Academy of Sciences; employed as Vice President of Food and Agriculture, Science and Regulatory Policy for the Biotechnology Industry Organization.

CLAYTON K. YEUTTER, past U.S. Department of Agriculture Secretary and United States trade representative. Member of the board of directors of Mycogen Seeds, whose majority owner is Dow Agro Sciences, a wholly owned subsidiary of the Dow Chemical Company.

LARRY ZEPH, former biologist of the EPA's Office of Prevention, Pesticides, and Toxic Substances; now Regulatory Science Manager at Pioneer Hi-Bred International, Inc.

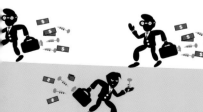
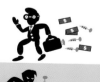

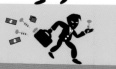
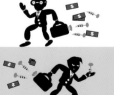
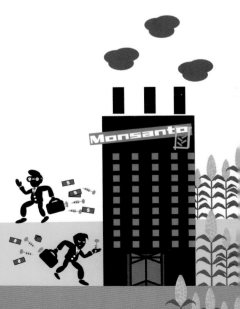

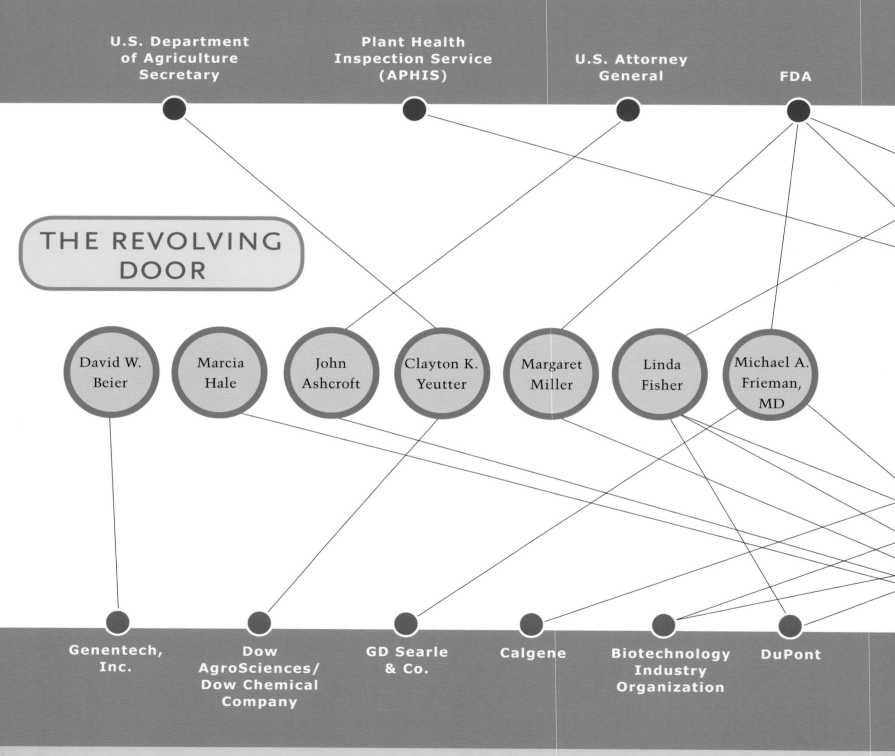

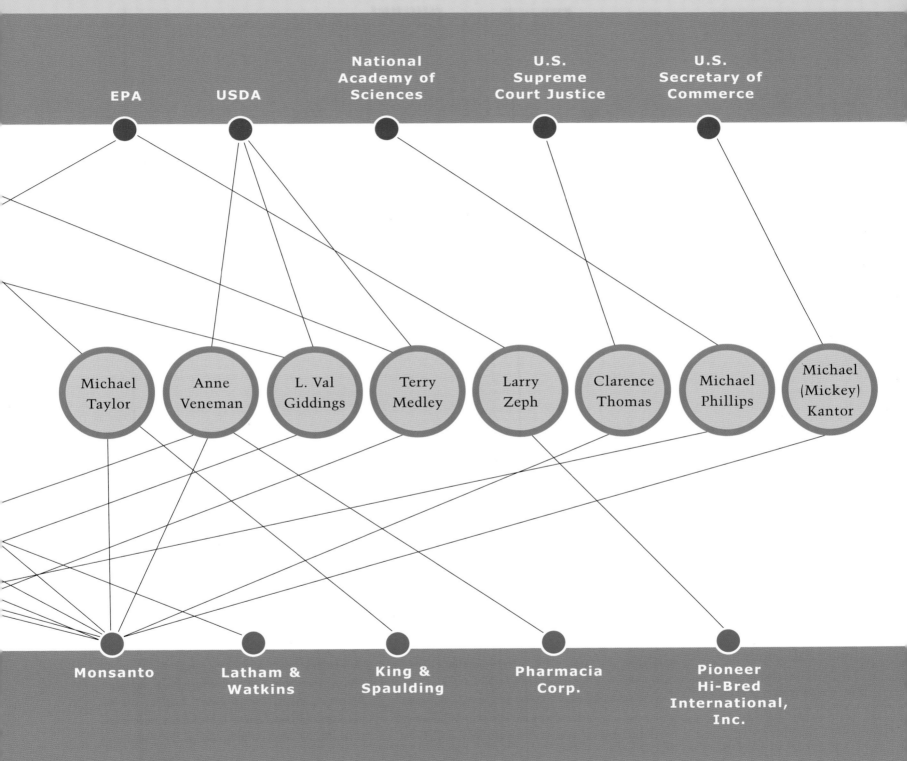

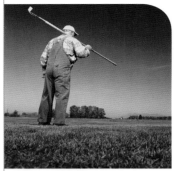

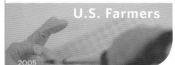

Monsanto vs.
U.S. Farmers

2005

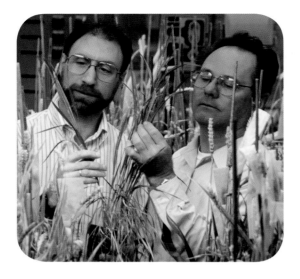

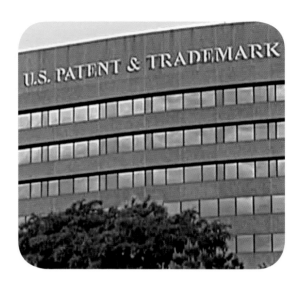

U.S. PATENT & TRADEMARK

Over the last few years, Monsanto has devoted significant resources to its prosecution of farmers who, like Percy Schmeiser, the company accuses of violating the company's seed patents. To investigate and pursue these alleged patent infringements, Monsanto created a legal department of seventy-five employees and set aside an annual budget of $10 million.[23] Monsanto says it receives hundreds of calls and letters each year about potential patent infringement cases. It also hires private investigation firms such as Robinson Investigations or Pinkerton to pursue growers suspected of illegally using its patented seeds. The investigators and other intimidation tactics often tear rural communities apart. For example, Monsanto advertises toll-free informer phone numbers in farm magazines across the country, encouraging farmers to turn in neighbors they suspect of saving patented GE seeds. Monsanto investigators wreak further damage by pitting neighbors against each other, offering reduced fines to growers who inform on fellow

farmers. The enormous penalties for planting patented seed—even when done so unintentionally—have forced numerous farmers into bankruptcy.

The full scope of Monsanto's patent inquisition is difficult to discern because the company's secret investigations far outnumber its publicly documented lawsuits. However, data gleaned from public sources reveal a disturbing picture. In 1998, Monsanto reported some 475 patent violation cases, generated from more than 1,800 leads nationwide.[24] In 1999, the *Washington Post* discovered 525 investigations in the United States and Canada.[25] Today, the annual number of investigations hovers between 500 and 600.[26] When the numbers are added up it is reasonable to conclude that over the last nine years, thousands of farmers have been investigated. Monsanto's persecution and prosecution of farmers often results in out-of-court settlements or litigation against farmers. Following investigations, Monsanto is known to send threatening

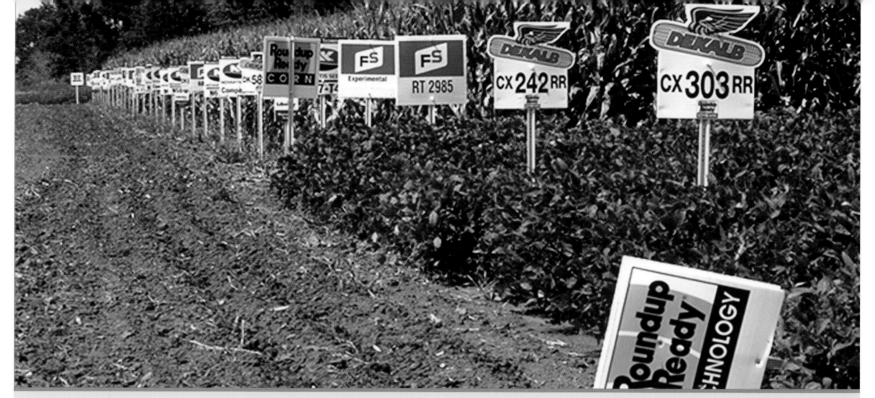

PATENTING LIFE: THE WORLD'S SEED MONOPOLY

TOP HOLDERS OF U.S. PATENTS IN AGRICULTURAL BIOTECHNOLOGY (INCLUDING SUBSIDIARIES)[27]

	Number of Patents		2004 Seed Sales (U.S. Millions)	Est. % of worldwide seed sales
1. Monsanto Co., Inc.	674	Monsanto (U.S.) + Seminis (acquired by Monsanto in 2005)	$2,277 + $526 pro forma = $2,803	13.3%
2. Du Pont, E.I. De Nemours & Co.	565	Dupont/Pioneer (U.S.)	$2,600	12.4%
3. Pioneer Hi-Bred International, Inc.	449	Syngenta (Switzerland)	$1,239	5.9%
4. U.S. Department Of Agriculture	315	Groupe Limagrain (France)	$1,044	5.0%
5. Syngenta	284	KWS AG (Germany)	$622	3.0%
6. Novartis Ag	230	Land O' Lakes (U.S.)	$538	2.6%
7. University Of California	221	Bayer Crop Science (Germany)	$387	2.0%
8. BASF Ag	217	Sakata (Japan)	$416	1.8%
9. Dow Chemical Co.	214	Taikii (Japan)	$366	1.7%
10. Hoechst Japan Ltd.	207	DLF-Trifolium (Denmark)	$320	1.5%
		Delta & Pine Land (U.S.)	$315	1.5%
		Top 2	$5,403	25.7%
		Top 5	$8,308	39.6%
		Top 11	$10,650	50.7%

Source: Adapted from ETC Group, Communiqué, Issue #90, Global Seed Industry Concentration — 2005.
http://www.etcgroup.org/documents/Comm90GlobalSeed.pdf

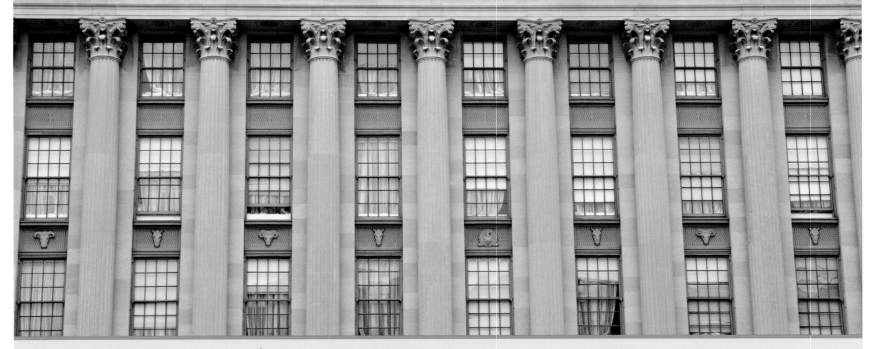

MONSANTO'S LAWSUITS AGAINST FARMERS FOR ALLEGED GE SEED-SAVING[28]

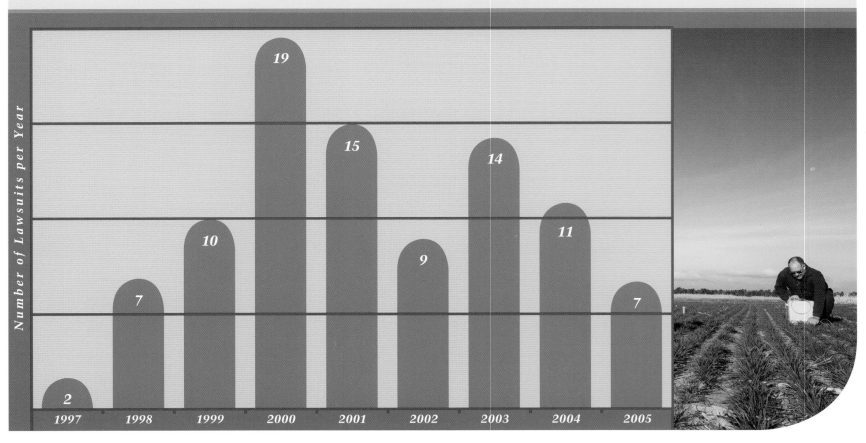

Number of Lawsuits per Year

1997	1998	1999	2000	2001	2002	2003	2004	2005
2	7	10	19	15	9	14	11	7

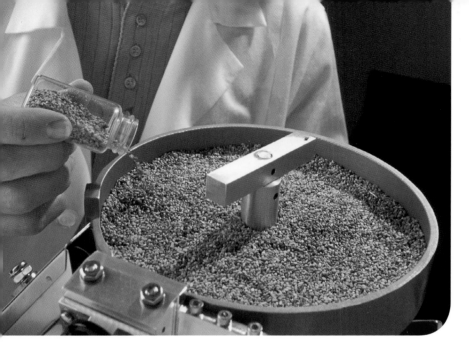

letters to growers suspected of planting or selling patented seed. These letters typically demand a specified sum of money to avoid legal proceedings. Monsanto also distributes literature to thousands of seed dealers each year, listing the names of farmers prohibited from purchasing its products. Under financial duress, many farmers accused of patent infringement based on insubstantial evidence decide to settle out of court instead of facing expensive and lengthy lawsuits.

Monsanto claims that since 2000, it has settled for millions of dollars in total damages.[29] Those unwilling to acquiesce to Monsanto's demands are vulnerable to aggressive litigation. Since 1997, Monsanto has filed more than ninety lawsuits based on purported violations of its technology agreement and its GE patents.[30] These cases have involved over 147 farmers and thirty-nine small businesses and farm companies.[31]

Monsanto, a multi-billion dollar company, unfairly presses cases against farmers who cannot afford good legal representation. Farmers sued by Monsanto often buckle under the additional expense of traveling to the company's corporate headquarters in St. Louis, Missouri, where they often must fight the lawsuit no matter where they farm. This keeps farmers at a disadvantage while increasing Monsanto's chances of a large payout.

Punitive damages along with auxiliary expenses—expert witness testimony, post-judgment interest, plaintiff's attorney costs and field-testing fees—can reach staggering proportions.

Fewer than half of the ninety judgments were publicly recorded; the majority of cases ended with confidential settlements. Of the judgments that are on record, the largest one made in Monsanto's favor was for $3,052,800. Monsanto's total reported awards for these lawsuits amount to $15,253,602; farmers pay a mean of $412,259 per case.[32]

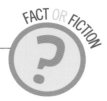

The U.S. government holds a patent on "Terminator technology" that makes plants sterile after a single growing season.

Fact In 1998, the USDA's Agricultural Research Service, together with Delta and Pine Land Company, received a patent entitled "Control of Plant Gene Expression." The patent covers GE technology that renders seeds sterile after a single growing season, thereby preventing farmers from saving them.[34]

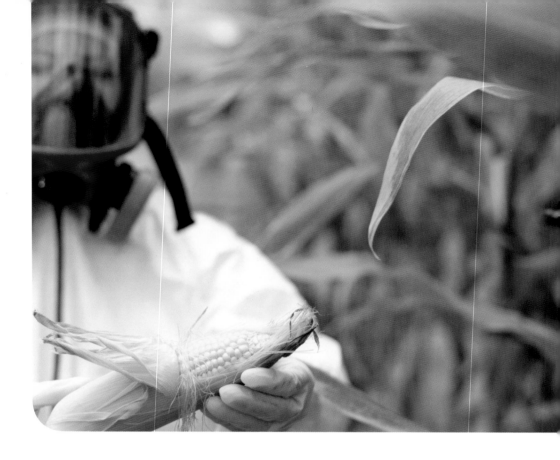

JUST SAYING NO

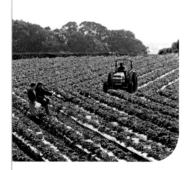

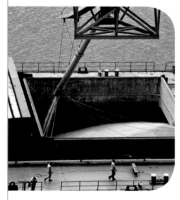

Faced with the devastating loss of the export and organic markets, angered by the persecution of farmers by companies like Monsanto, more and more growers are saying no to GE crops. As recently as 2004, Monsanto was poised to commercialize its GE wheat, but a powerful grassroots effort led by farmers in the Dakotas and Montana forced the company to abandon its plans. Meanwhile, rice farmers in California and in other regions have thwarted biotech endeavors to commercialize GE rice. Farmers around the country have also protested the use of GE crops to produce vaccines and other chemicals—so-called "biopharmaceuticals." Their campaigns have successfully persuaded major biotech conglomerates to abandon the development and testing of these crops.

Michael Sligh, of The Rural Advancement Foundation International, sums up the situation: "Farmers in this country and around the world are increasingly organizing to protect themselves and their communities from the devastating impacts of genetic engineering and the companies that promote it. We will not allow our markets to be lost and our right to save our seeds undermined. We know our future lies with sustainable and socially just farming practices and not with technologies and patent policies that only profit a few corporations."

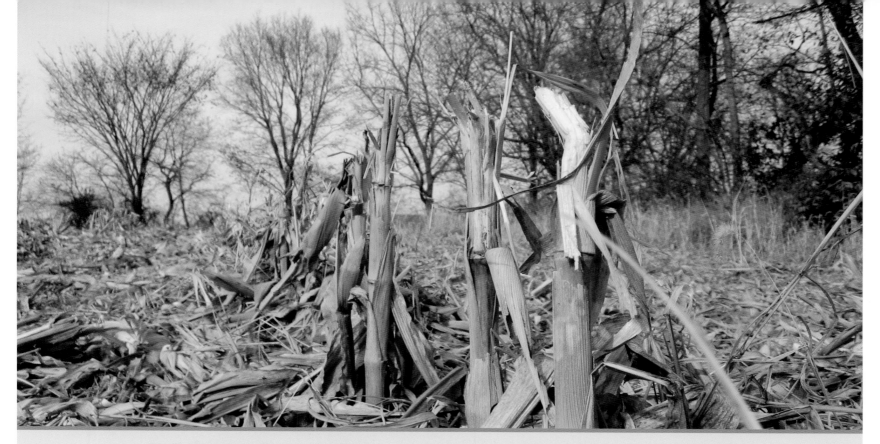

TERMINATOR TECHNOLOGY: THE "SUICIDE GENE" FOR PLANTS

What is Terminator technology?

"Terminator technology" refers to plants that have been genetically engineered to produce sterile seed; that is, to "commit suicide" after one growing season. Terminator was developed by the biotech industry and the U.S. government to prevent farmers from re-planting harvested seed and to maximize seed industry profits; the USDA, Delta & Pine Land, Syngenta, DuPont, BASF, and Monsanto all hold patents on Terminator. Terminator plants have not yet been commercialized or field-tested—although trials are currently being conducted in greenhouses in the U.S.

Why is Terminator a problem?

Over 1.4 billion people, primarily small-scale farming families in the developing world, depend on farm-saved seed as their primary seed source. Since Terminator seeds are sterile after one growing season there is no use in saving them. The widespread use and dissemination of Terminator seeds or mixing of them with conventional seed will mean that these hundreds of millions of farmers could be forced one day to buy seeds each year from corporations like Monsanto as some or all of their own seeds commit suicide each year. This could bankrupt these farmers and disrupt indigenous peoples' seed exchange practices, creating food shortages and increasing starvation around the world. Additionally, Terminator technology destroys the age-old practice of farmer seed selection and breeding—the foundation for local seed security.

To learn more, visit www.banterminator.org

> "I have held in my hand the germ of a plant engineered to grow, yield its crop, and then murder its own embryos, and there I glimpsed the malevolence that can lie in the heart of a profiteering enterprise."
>
> —*Barbara Kingsolver*
> *Author*

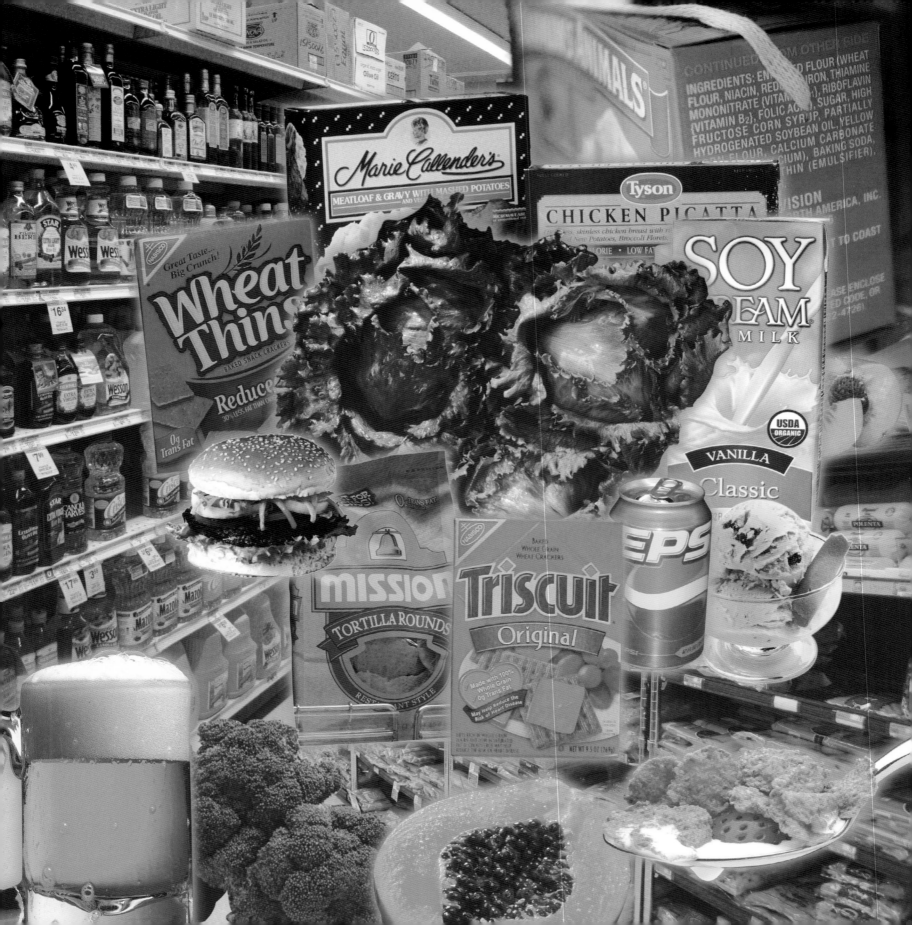

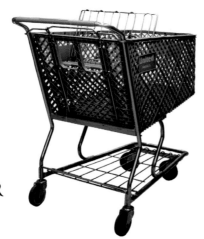

CHAPTER FOUR

A Quick Guide to Genetically Engineered Foods in Your Supermarket

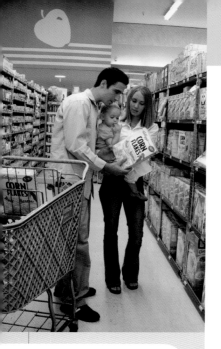

Reclaim your right to know about the foods you are buying. This guide will help you identify the GE foods that are lurking in your supermarket.

Our government, under pressure from the biotechnology industry, has not required the labeling of GE foods.

Which supermarket foods are genetically engineered? This is probably the most urgent question the public has about these novel foods. Opinion polls show that up to 90 percent of the American public wants GE foods labeled. But despite this overwhelming demand, almost no foods on U.S. grocery shelves reveal their secret, genetically engineered ingredients.

We've seen that our government, under pressure from the biotechnology industry, has not required the labeling of GE foods. And the biotech industry does not voluntarily identify them, fearing, probably correctly, that the majority of Americans would avoid GE foods if given a choice. As a result, the U.S. public has been deprived of its right to choose whether to buy and consume these engineered foods. However, this is not the case with most of our major trading partners around the globe who have instituted mandatory labeling of all GE foods and ingredients.[1]

This Quick Guide is designed as an accessible way for you to reclaim your right to know about the foods you are buying. It will help you identify the GE foods that are in your supermarket. Rather than provide you with a long and unmanageable list of brands and products, the guide offers you easy-to-follow advice for each area of your supermarket. These tips will help you find and avert GE foods and ingredients.

For those interested in detailed information, we also include in Appendix 1 a more in-depth shopping list, where we identify the leading brands of packaged foods, snacks, and other products that may contain GE ingredients. We also list non-GE alternatives you can purchase. With this information in hand, you can shop with confidence, knowing that you won't unwittingly expose your family to the hazards of GE food.

SHOPPING OVERVIEW

It's helpful, when trying to identify GE food in your supermarket, to keep three general categories of food in mind: 1) Products in your supermarket that are not genetically engineered and contain no genetically engineered ingredients; 2) Food made from animals that are not genetically engineered, but may have been raised on genetically engineered feed or treated with genetically engineered hormones; and 3) Whole foods that are genetically engineered or processed foods that are likely to contain genetically engineered ingredients.

1) Foods that have not been genetically engineered

Fortunately, avoiding many genetically engineered foods is simple. For example, most whole foods for sale—almost all fruits and vegetables as well as staples such as rice, wheat, and other grains and beans—are not genetically engineered. You can purchase these foods and products without concern.

2) Foods derived from animals fed or treated with GE products

The good news is GE animals, including fish, are not commercialized. So you can purchase these products without the fear of genetic tampering; furthermore, this guide will also help you identify and avoid meat, fish, and dairy products derived from animals that have been fed or treated with GE products. This includes processed foods that possibly contain milk-derived ingredients, like whey and milk powders or solids, from cows given the GE hormone rbGH (or rbST).

3) Genetically engineered foods and ingredients

Unfortunately, certain widely used crops have been genetically altered. Of most concern are the "Big Four": corn, soy, canola, and cotton. Today, an estimated 52 percent of all corn, 87 percent of all soy 55 percent of all canola, and 79 percent of all cotton grown in the U.S. are genetically engineered.[2] These Big Four GE crops—especially their byproducts— find their way into the majority of packaged foods in our supermarkets. Some of the most common genetically engineered Big Four ingredients in processed foods are

- **Corn:** corn oil, corn meal, cornstarch, corn syrup
- **Soy:** soybean oil, soy flour, soy protein, soy lecithin
- **Canola:** canola oil
- **Cotton:** cottonseed oil

As you will see throughout this Quick Guide, a major rule when recognizing and ducking GE foods is to "Beware the Big Four" and their byproducts.

START THE SUPERMARKET TOUR

Now that you have an overview of GE foods it's time to take a tour around your supermarket aisles where we'll provide you with specific advice on identifying GE foods and ingredients. As we visit each major supermarket section, you'll learn important tips on singling out—and sidestepping—GE foods.

Labels can give you detailed information—above and beyond the fat and carbohydrate contents—about the food you eat. But you have to know how to decode the language. Below, you'll find some helpful tips on deciphering the word "organic," and how it's applied to the food you buy.

What is organic food?

The International Federation of Organic Agricultural Movements (IFOAM) defines organic food production as a "holistic production management system which promotes and enhances agro-ecosystem health, including biodiversity, biological cycles, and soil biological activity. [Organic food production] excludes the use of synthetic inputs, such as synthetic fertilizers and pesticides, veterinary drugs, genetically modified seeds and breeds, preservatives, additives, and irradiation." You can learn more about organic food at www.ifoam.org/organic_facts/index.html.

What are "Organic" labels?

Under U.S. Department of Agriculture policy, genetically engineered seed cannot be used in organic production.[3] Four types of labels are allowed on organic foods. See the agency's explanation at www.ams.usda.gov/nop/ProdHandlers/labelTable.htm

1. Foods labeled "100% organic" are single foods, usually fruits or vegetables, which have been grown organically, or packaged foods with all-organic ingredients.

2. The word "organic" on the front of packaged foods means that organic ingredients comprise at least 95 percent of the product.

3. Foods can be labeled "with organic (ingredients)" if they are at least 70 percent organic.

4. Packaged foods manufactured with less than 70 percent of organic ingredients may list the ingredients as "organic" on the side-panel ingredient list, but cannot use "organic" on the front of the package. Organic foods are certified by independent, third-party, organic-standards organizations and governed by federal rules set by the USDA.

Labels like "natural," "free-range" and "hormone-free" are not subject to organic standards, unless they are also labeled "organic." For most foods, there are no standards for products labeled "natural," so check the ingredients list as carefully as you would any other product for non-organic corn, soy, canola, or cottonseed oil that may be genetically engineered.

What are "GE-Free" labels?

Manufacturers have been active in creating a market for GE-free foods. According to an April 2006 USDA report, from 2000 to 2004, manufacturers introduced over 3,500 products that had non-GE labeling. Although these products are not subject to third-party verifed standards (as is the organic label), they show that manufacturers are increasingly sourcing non-GE ingredients in their food products.

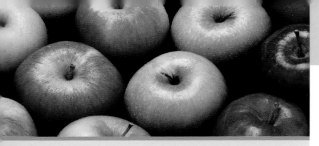

FRUITS & VEGETABLES

Fortunately, very few fresh fruits and vegetables for sale in the U.S. are genetically engineered. Papaya is the main exception (see below). Additionally, gene-altered sweet corn, zucchini, and some summer squash varieties do occasionally crop up in stores, but it's rare.

Quick Hints—conventional

•Most GE papaya is grown in Hawaii, where about half of papayas are genetically engineered.[5] Consumers on the West Coast may want to check with their supermarket produce manager to see whether or not the papaya sold at that market is genetically engineered. Outside of the West Coast, most of the papaya you'll find comes from countries like Brazil and Mexico and areas like the Caribbean, where GE varieties are not cultivated.[6]

•Most GE soy and corn become animal feed; the vast majority of the remainder is incorporated into processed foods. Finding GE sweet corn in the fresh produce section is rare, but if you are concerned, ask your grocer to find out from their suppliers.

•Although infrequent, GE squash (zucchini, yellow crookneck squash), is grown in small amounts; ask your grocer if you are concerned.

Quick Hints—organic

•To be sure your food is non-GE, buy certified organic summer squash, sweet corn, and papaya.

> **FACT**
> Fortunately, very few fresh fruits and vegetables for sale in the U.S. are genetically engineered.

"How we eat determines, to a considerable extent, how the world is used."[7]

—*Wendell Berry*
Author, poet, and farmer

PEACE OF MIND

Despite the general misconception that GE contamination is widespread, the vast majority of fruits, vegetables, and grains on the market are still GE-free. Enjoy these foods—sold in your favorite store—with peace of mind:

Apples	Cucumbers	Peaches
Asparagus	Honey	Pears
Avocados	Lemons	Peas
Bananas	Lettuce	Peppers
Beets	Maple Syrup	Pineapple
Berries	Molasses	Potatoes
Broccoli	Mushrooms	Rice
Grapes	Nuts	Spinach
Cane Sugar	Oats	Tomatoes
Carrots	Olives	Watermelons
Celery	Onions	Wheat
	Oranges	

DID YOU KNOW?

Voluntary stickers on produce can provide clues about whether an item is organic, conventional, or genetically engineered.

According to the International Federation of Produce Coding, Price Look-up codes—the numbers found on the round stickers on produce—can indicate the way in which a piece of produce was grown.[4] Since the system is voluntary, the codes are not a foolproof guide, but they still may be a valuable source of information.

Conventionally grown
4-digit code

Organically grown
5-digit code starting in 9

Genetically engineered
5-digit code starting in 8

MEATS & FISH

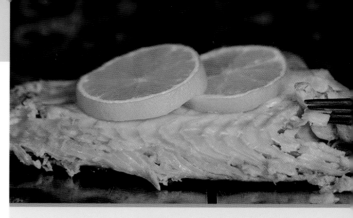

You'll be glad to know that thanks to the hard work of many food and farming organizations, no genetically engineered fish, fowl, or livestock is yet approved for human consumption. However, plenty of food is produced from animals raised on GE feed such as grains. You may still want to stay away from these items.

Quick Hints—conventional

•To avoid meat raised on genetically engineered feed crops, look for the phrase "100% grass fed."

•Processed and precooked meat and fish may contain genetically engineered oil-based additives and preservatives. Canned tuna may be packed in GE oils; to be safe, buy canned fish packed in water or olive oil.

•Farm-grown fish (trout, catfish, salmon) can be raised on genetically engineered feed. Look for wild rather than farmed fish to avoid this possibility.

Quick Hints—organic ∿

•Look for certified organic chicken, beef, pork, and processed meat or fish products.

FACT ‹

No genetically engineered fish, fowl, or livestock is yet approved for human consumption.

"It is important that citizens let the government know how they feel about genetically engineered food. I have concerns that this untested technology diminishes the purity and taste of food."[8]

—*Charlie Trotter*
1999 James Beard Chef of the Year

SHOP SMART, SHOP HEALTHY:

Wise Choices at the Meat and Seafood Counters
For a directory on sustainably raised meats, poultry and eggs, visit the Institute for Agriculture and Trade Policy's Eat Well Guide: www.eatwellguide.org

To learn more about genetically engineered fish, visit:

www.centerforfoodsafety.org/geneticall3.cfm

For a printable guide to seafood, visit:
www.mbayaq.org/cr/cr_seafoodwatch/download.asp

Although this guide from the Monterey Bay Aquarium talks about the many concerns of farm-raised fish, it does not specifically address the issue of GE feed in farmed-fish operations. Nevertheless, the guide will give you a good starting point in deciding what fish to buy. Also check out the Center for Food Safety's guide to aquaculture, "The Catch with Seafood," available on CFS's website, www.centerforfoodsafety.org.

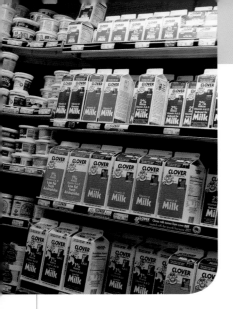

IN THE DAIRY CASE

MILK PRODUCTS

The good news is that dairy products from GE cows are not approved for commercial sale. However, the diet of most dairy cows likely includes genetically engineered grains. Also, some U.S. dairy farms inject the genetically engineered hormone rbGH, also called rbST, into their cows to boost milk production. To steer clear of genetic engineering in the dairy section, follow these hints below.

Quick Hints—conventional

Look for dairy products labeled "100% grass-fed."

Find products with a label that indicates cows free of rbGH or rbST. On some brands, the label will say "no artificial hormones."

Sheep and goats are not administered rbGH.

Many yogurts contain corn syrup as a sweetener. To avoid GE corn syrup, seek yogurts sweetened with sugar, natural fruit, honey, or pure maple syrup.

Quick Hints—organic ❧

Certified organic dairy products are guaranteed to come from cows not administered rbGH or raised on GE feed.

ALTERNATIVE DAIRY PRODUCTS

Buying alternative dairy products is an easy way to skirt some of the problems associated with dairy factory farming, which uses rbGH and genetically engineered feed. Since many alternatives are made from soybeans, and 87 percent of soy is genetically engineered,[10] many of these products may contain GE materials. Consequently, many companies are responding to consumer concerns by providing GE-free non-dairy products.

Quick Hints—conventional

To stay GE-free, consider beverages and foods made from rice or nut milk— keep in mind that additives and sweeteners can be derived from GE crops. Check for GE-free labels on some of these products.

Quick Hints—organic ❧

To ensure your soy milk is GE-free, buy certified organic products.

Beware: Soy milk can list "organic soybeans" as an ingredient but may still contain other ingredients or additives formulated from GE crops. Check for the USDA "organic" seal on the front of the package.

EGGS

Right now, no genetically engineered egg-laying chickens are on the market. Nevertheless, non-organic, egg-producing chickens eat genetically modified grains such as corn and soy.

Quick Hints—conventional

Beware: Eggs labeled "free-range," "free-roaming," "natural," or "cage-free" are not guaranteed to be GE-free.[11]

Quick Hints—organic ❧

Look for certified organic eggs.

Your Right to Know 84

DID YOU KNOW?

Dairy products bearing the Maine Quality Trademark have been produced without the use of recombinant bovine growth hormone (rbGH).

To use Maine's red, white, and blue seal for quality, a producer must supply a statement that "the applicant believes that the milk the applicant has or will purchase or produce is from cows not treated with rbST."[9] (rbST is another term for rbGH.) Look out for this seal on your New England dairy products.

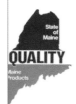

State of Maine

QUALITY
Maine Products

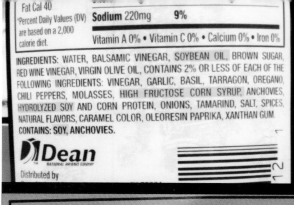

Fat Cal 40
*Percent Daily Values (DV) are based on a 2,000 calorie diet.
Sodium 220mg 9%
Vitamin A 0% • Vitamin C 0% • Calcium 0% • Iron 0%

INGREDIENTS: WATER, BALSAMIC VINEGAR, SOYBEAN OIL, BROWN SUGAR, RED WINE VINEGAR, VIRGIN OLIVE OIL, CONTAINS 2% OR LESS OF EACH OF THE FOLLOWING INGREDIENTS: VINEGAR, GARLIC, BASIL, TARRAGON, OREGANO, CHILI PEPPERS, MOLASSES, HIGH FRUCTOSE CORN SYRUP, ANCHOVIES, HYDROLYZED SOY AND CORN PROTEIN, ONIONS, TAMARIND, SALT, SPICES, NATURAL FLAVORS, CARAMEL COLOR, OLEORESIN PAPRIKA, XANTHAN GUM. CONTAINS: SOY, ANCHOVIES.

Dean
NATIONAL BRAND GROUP
Distributed by

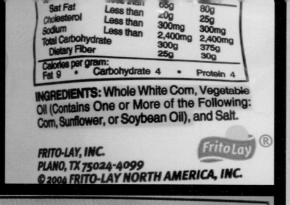

INGREDIENTS: Whole White Corn, Vegetable Oil (Contains One or More of the Following: Corn, Sunflower, or Soybean Oil), and Salt.

FRITO-LAY, INC.
PLANO, TX 75024-4099
© 2004 FRITO-LAY NORTH AMERICA, INC.

FritoLay ®

Potassium ... Less than 2,400mg 2,400mg
3,500mg 3,500mg
Total Carbohydrate 300g 375g
Dietary Fiber 25g 30g
Calories per gram: Fat 9 • Carbohydrate 4 • Protein 4

Ingredients: Milled corn, sugar, malt flavoring, high fructose corn syrup, salt,

Vitamins and Iron: Iron, niacinamide, sodium ascorbate and ascorbic acid (vitamin C), pyridoxine hydrochloride (vitamin B6), riboflavin (vitamin B2), thiamin hydrochloride (vitamin B1), vitamin A palmitate, folic acid, vitamin B12 and vitamin D. To maintain quality, BHT has been added to the packaging.

CORN USED IN THIS PRODUCT CONTAINS TRACES OF SOYBEANS.

Exchange: 1½ Carbohydrates
The dietary exchanges are based on the *Exchange Lists for Meal Planning,* ©2003 by The American Diabetes Association, Inc. and The American Dietetic Association.

INGREDIENTS: TOMATO CONCENTRATE (WATER AND TOMATO PASTE), HIGH FRUCTOSE CORN SYRUP, CORN SYRUP, VINEGAR, SALT, ONION POWDER, SPICE, NATURAL FLAVORS.

DISTRIBUTED BY
SAFEWAY INC.
P.O. BOX 99, PLEASANTON, CA 94566-0009
1-888-SAFEWAY / www.safeway.com
PRODUCT OF U.S.A.

HIDDEN GE INGREDIENTS

Processed foods typically contain ingredients derived from the Big Four GE crops, especially corn and soy. But these secret derivatives are often undercover behind complex or ambiguous names. Some of these derivatives are also created using GE microorganisms. Look out for the common ingredients listed below, and remember that the surest way to avoid GE-derived ingredients in processed foods is to buy certified organic.

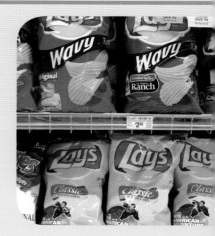

Corn
- Corn flour, meal, oil, starch, gluten, and syrup
- Sweeteners such as fructose, dextrose, and glucose*
- Food starch and modified food starch*
- Mono- and diglycerides*
- Vitamin C (ascorbic acid)*

Canola
- Canola oil (also called rapeseed oil)

Soybeans
- Soy flour, lecithin, protein, oil, isolate, and isoflavones
- Vegetable oil*
- Vegetable protein*
- Vitamin E (tocopherols)*

Cotton
- Cottonseed oil

* May be derived from other sources

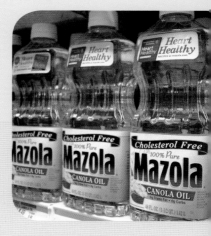

Sources: "Non-Organic Ingredients Provide Pathway for GMOs in Organic Foods," *The Non-GMO Report*, Vol. 6, Issue 3, March 2006.

"Genetically Engineered Foods In the Marketplace," Cornell Cooperative Extension's Genetically Engineered Organisms Public Issues in Education (GEO-PIE) Project, last updated May 2003.

BABY FOODS

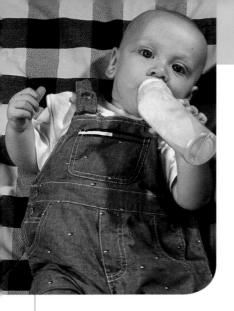

Most foods for infants are just what the label says with few preservatives or additives except water. You can puree fresh fruits and veggies (except non-organic papaya, yellow squash, corn, or soy) daily for your baby, or try preparing a large batch and freezing it in small jars, bags, ice-trays or containers to thaw and use later. This gives you the ease of portable, serving-sized jars, and lets you know exactly what's in it because you made it! If you can't puree fresh products on a daily basis, try these suggestions:

Quick Hints—conventional

Some baby cereals can have GE ingredients even if the primary component is GE-free. For example, some rice cereals add soy lecithin as an emulsifier, which can be processed from GE soy. Look for cereals with one or a few ingredients, or make your own. Buy a new coffee grinder. Grind rice and other grains for simple, homemade baby cereals.

Teething crackers and biscuits can contain GE corn syrup and soy lecithin.

Food for older babies and toddlers, such as noodles and cheese, often contain processed ingredients derived from genetically engineered sources.

These days even some non-organic brands such as Gerber have pledged to avoid GE ingredients in all of their baby foods.

Quick Hints—organic ∿

Certified organic brands are sure to be free of GE ingredients.

INFANT FORMULA

Milk or soy protein is the basis of most infant formulas. The secret ingredients in these products are often soy or milk from cows injected with rbGH. Many brands also add GE-derived corn syrup or corn syrup solids.

Quick Hints—organic ∿

If you can't breastfeed, or need to supplement, buy certified organic infant formulas or formulas labeled GE-free.

[Note throughout: Not all GE-free products are certified organic.]

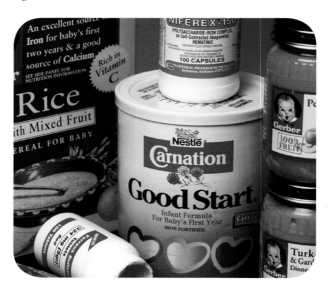

GRAINS & BEANS

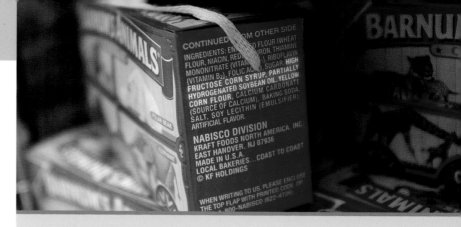

Fortunately, circumventing genetically modified food in the grain-and-bean aisle is simple. Other than corn, no GE grains are sold on the market. Most pasta is made from a few ingredients. As long as you avoid the less-common corn pasta, you're in the clear. Likewise, dried beans are often just beans with no additives.

Quick Hints—conventional

Look for 100-percent wheat pasta, couscous, rice, quinoa, oats, barley, sorghum, and dried beans (except soybeans).

Watch out for additives and other potential GE ingredients in the seasoning packets of boxed pasta and rice-based meals.

Quick Hints—organic ∾

Choose certified organic brands or GE-free brands of corn pasta, soybeans, and polenta.

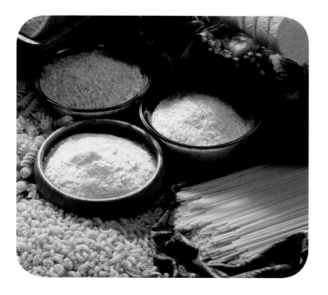

TOP TEN CHILDREN'S FOODS CONTAINING GE INGREDIENTS

Listed below are conventionally produced children's foods. Non-organic versions of these popular foods may contain GE ingredients, as noted.

1. Hot dogs: soy protein, meat, milk produced from animals fed GE corn and soy, milk treated with rbGH.

2. Macaroni and cheese: canola and soy oils, milk produced from animals treated with rbGH.

3. Breakfast cereal: corn, corn syrup, soy and canola oils, soy lecithin.

4. Chips: soybean, corn, canola and cottonseed oils, corn, corn starch, corn syrup.

5. Tomato sauce: canola and soybean oils, corn syrup.

6. French fries: canola, soybean and corn oils.

7. Ice cream: corn syrup, milk produced from animals treated with rBGH, cottonseed and soybean oils, soy lecithin.

8. Soda: corn syrup.

9. Peanut butter: corn syrup, soybean and canola oils, soy lecithin.

10. Granola Bars: soybean, cottonseed and canola oils, milk produced from animals treated with rbGH, soy lecithin, corn syrup, soy protein.

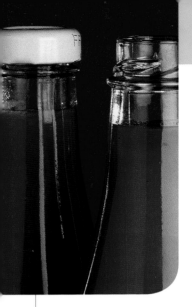

CONDIMENTS, OILS, DRESSINGS, AND SPREADS

Fortunately, plenty of healthy, non-GE options are available in this category (see below). Unless labeled explicitly, corn, soybean, cottonseed, and canola oils probably contain genetically engineered products. Ketchup usually incorporates corn syrup; and mayonnaise and most conventional salad dressings use soy, cottonseed, or canola oil as a major ingredient. Many creamy dressings and sauces will also include milk solids or powders, which may be derived from cows treated with rbGH or rbST. Instead, look for products sweetened with pure maple syrup, honey, molasses, or pure cane sugar rather than corn syrups.

Quick Hints—conventional

Choose pure olive, coconut, sesame, sunflower, safflower, almond, and peanut oils (not products mixed with canola, soy, cottonseed, or corn oil).

Look for preserves, jams, and jellies with sugar, not corn syrup.

Look for conventional nut butters without added soy, corn, cottonseed, or canola oil.

Quick Hints—organic ∾

Choose products identified as "certified organic" or labeled "GE-free."

SOUPS AND SAUCES

Shopping for soups and sauces can be challenging. Many are highly processed and include ingredients that can be genetically engineered. Pay close attention to the ingredient lists and, when possible, stick to certified organic and GE-free labeled brands.

Quick Hints—conventional

Think simple. The fewer ingredients and flavors a product contains, the less likely it is to harbor genetically engineered components.

Quick Hints—organic ∾

Choose certified organic brands and GE-free brands.

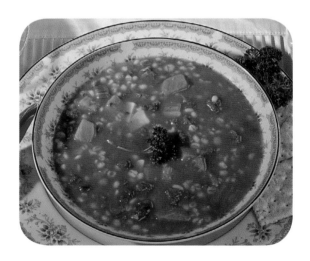

"The choices we make when we buy food are serious choices... When people choose organic foods and avoid mass-produced and fast foods, they are voting for a sustainable future and against a network of supply and demand that destroys human health, local communities, traditional ways of life, and the environment."[12]

—*Alice Waters*
Chef, Chez Panisse restaurant

CANNED & FROZEN FOODS

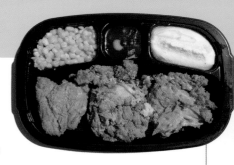

CANNED FOODS

Finding GE-free vegetables, beans, tomatoes, and seafood is easy; however, canned goods that are flavored or highly processed offer more of a challenge. When shopping for canned fruits and meats and flavored sauces, look for items marked "certified organic" and brands that don't contain potential GE ingredients. Remember to watch out for the Big Four GE crops—corn, soy, canola, and cottonseed—and their derivatives.

Quick Hints—conventional

Search for canned vegetable/bean/tomato products packed only in water and salt.

Common GE ingredients in canned foods are: corn syrup; corn, soy, canola, and cottonseed oils; and cornstarch.

Other good choices are plain beans (except soybeans) packed in water; plain vegetables (except corn) packed in water; stewed or crushed tomatoes; 100-percent tomato paste; seafood packed in its own juices, water or olive oil; and mixed vegetables (excluding corn).

Many flavored or extra-processed products (baked beans, flavored tomato sauces, canned meats) can contain GE ingredients.

Additionally, some canned and flavored tomato sauces contain the Big Four ingredients.

Quick Hints—organic

As always, look for certified organic brands and GMO-free brands.

FROZEN FOODS

Many frozen foods are highly processed. When choosing foods from the freezer aisle, check the label to see whether or not the product contains genetically altered ingredients. Keep an eye out for the Big Four and stay away from frozen foods that contain them, unless they are marked organic or non-GE. Luckily, many frozen vegetables and fruits don't have any other additives, making these products good choices.

Quick Hints—conventional

Choose plain frozen fruits and veggies (except for non-organic squash and corn) that do not contain other ingredients that may be GE.

Quick Hints—organic

Look for certified organic frozen dishes and foods labeled "GMO- or GE-Free."

Watch out for products containing non-organic soy, corn, canola, or cottonseed.

> "Mother Nature has done a great job on her own. Genetic engineers are creating substances the body has never experienced. These foods cannot be as healthful as natural foods, and they certainly cannot be as flavorful in cooking."[13]
>
> —*Rick Moonen*
> *Chef, rm restaurant*

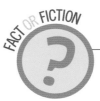

More than fifty countries require the labeling of GE foods.

Fact At least fifty-one countries around the world require some labeling of GE foods, including the entire European Union, Australia, New Zealand, Brazil, Chile, India, China, and Japan.[14]

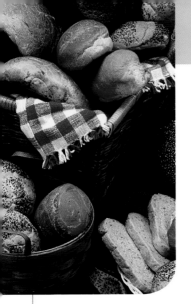

FACT
Pressure from farmers and consumers forced Monsanto to shelve its plans to introduce genetically engineered wheat into the market.

BREAD, BAKED GOODS, and BAKING SUPPLIES

Pressure from farmers and consumers has forced Monsanto to shelve its plans to introduce genetically engineered wheat into the market. Because wheat is a major ingredient in most baked goods, GE-free bakery products are easier to find than some other foods. Nevertheless, many packaged breads and bakery items contain other GE ingredients, so the best way to avoid genetically engineered baked goods is—you guessed it—to buy organic.

Quick Hints—conventional

Stay away from breads, baked goods, and baking mixes made with soy; corn syrup; and corn, canola, or cottonseed oil.

Baking ingredients such as wheat flour, rice, kamut, and oats are not genetically engineered.

Ask the in-store baker if he or she uses GE ingredients.

If you're baking sweetened breads and other treats that call for a syrup, use a non-corn syrup sweetener like honey, pure maple syrup, or molasses.

Quick Hints—organic

Many conventional chocolate chips and baking chocolates contain corn syrup and soy lecithin, which are often GE ingredients. Milk and white chocolate varieties may contain milk-derived ingredients from cows treated with rbGH. Look for certified organic or non-GE brands.

Corn meal, starch, and syrup may be made from GE corn; ask your supplier about their policies or buy organic. Baking powder, which contains corn starch, can also be derived from GE corn; search for organic or non-GE baking powder.

CEREALS and BREAKFAST BARS

Cereals and breakfast bars are very likely to include genetically engineered ingredients because they are often made with corn and soy products.

Quick Hints—conventional

Choose cereals that are made from wheat, rice, or oatmeal and sweetened with honey, pure maple syrup, molasses or sugar, not corn syrup.

Quick Hints—organic

Cereals marked "GMO-free," "GE-free," and "certified organic" are fine.

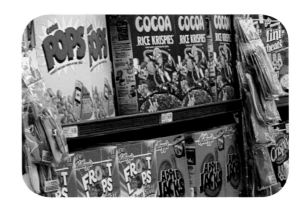

SNACK FOOD

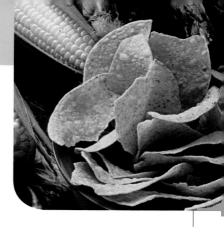

SNACKS

Many snack foods contain ingredients acquired from the Big Four genetically engineered crops. These ingredients may comprise a large part of the food, like the corn in corn chips, or they may play a more minor role, like the soy lecithin in a cookie. Snack foods, because of their many ingredients, can seem like a minefield of GE products. Fortunately, there are GE-free options.

Quick Hints—conventional

Look for snacks made from wheat, rice, or oats, along with other non-GE ingredients.

Nuts and seeds (such as peanuts and sunflower seeds) and dried fruits (such as raisins) are good GE-free options.

Watch out for non-organic snacks that contain corn, soy, canola, cottonseed, or any of their derivatives; these tend to be found as oils, sweeteners, and preservatives.

Snacks labeled "natural" are not necessarily GE-free.[16]

Quick Hints—organic ∾

Buy snack foods labeled or similarly identified as "certified organic," "GMO-free," or "Made without genetically engineered ingredients."

CHOCOLATE PRODUCTS and CANDY

Most conventional chocolates contain corn syrup and soy lecithin, the two popular GE additives. Milk chocolate products are often manufactured with milk from cows treated with rbGH. Most candy also contains corn syrup, soy lecithin, and other ingredients derived from corn or soy. Sugar-free candies often contain aspartame, known commercially as NutraSweet. NutraSweet can be made from genetically modified crops.

Quick Hints—conventional

Watch out for ingredients such as soy lecithin, corn syrup, and other ingredients derived from the Big Four: corn, soy, canola, and cottonseed.

Quick Hints—organic ∾

As always, certified organic candy or candy labeled "GMO- or GE-Free" will not contain GE ingredients.

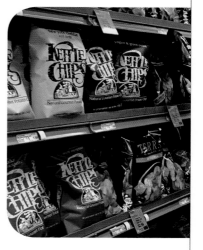

DID YOU KNOW?

Popcorn is not genetically engineered.

According to the U.S. Popcorn Board, "There is no genetically modified popcorn (kernels) currently available for sale in domestic or international markets."[17] Furthermore, decades before the advent of GE, popcorn was bred not to cross with other kinds of corn.[18] This means that accidental contamination of popcorn with GE is less likely than for other kinds of corn. At least for now, this snack is GE-free.

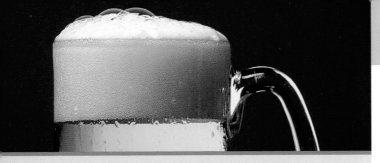

BUD VS. COORS: BEER-MAKERS WEIGH IN ON GENETICALLY ENGINEERED CROPS

While there are currently no genetically engineered ingredients in beer, two beer-makers have taken very different stances on the use of biotech crops in beer: Budweiser has helped put the brakes on a field trial of biopharmaceutical rice in Missouri. Having worn out its welcome in California, a biotech company, Ventria, took its plan to test genetically engineered, "biopharmaceutical" rice to Missouri, Anheuser-Busch's back yard. Ventria probably didn't guess that a beer behemoth would get in its way. But Anheuser-Busch wouldn't stand by and allow for the possibility that drug-producing rice could commingle with the rice it uses to make beer. The company's vice president stated that "[g]iven the potential for contamination of commercial rice production in this state, we will not purchase any rice produced or processed in Missouri if Ventria introduces its pharma rice here."[19] The company later modified its stance given the stringent confinement of the trial, but by that time, Ventria had already gone packing to North Carolina.

In contrast to Budweiser, the Coors Brewing Company, which often relies on its image of Rocky Mountain purity, has gone gung-ho for genetically engineering its product. Coors has established a strategic alliance with a Sacramento, California biotechnological company called Applied Phytologics Inc. (API). The stated purpose of Coors' alliance with API is "to develop and commercialize genetically engineered grains to improve the malting process..." What's worse, the Center for Food Safety discovered through a Freedom of Information Act request to the USDA that Coors has been receiving hundreds of grams of genetically engineered wheat seeds from API and planting it in field trials. Whether this wheat has already contaminated conventional wheat or entered the food chain is unknown.

BEVERAGES

The good news is, since papaya is the only whole fruit that is genetically engineered, most juices are made from GE-free fruit. On the other hand, the prevalence of corn-based sweeteners in fruit juices is cause for concern. Similarly many sodas are primarily comprised of water and corn syrup—there is a high probability that these drinks contain genetically engineered ingredients.

Quick Hints – conventional

Look for 100-percent juice blends (except those containing papaya juice).

Buy beverages sweetened with sugar rather than corn syrup or aspartame.

Keep an eye out for corn syrup and high-fructose corn syrup in children's drink mixes, juice boxes, and drink pouches.

Unsweetened drinks and products sweetened with fruit, cane juice, cane sugar, honey, or other non-corn ingredients are safe.

Tart juices like cranberry or grapefruit most likely contain a sweetener, while juices made from naturally sweet fruits such as apples or oranges are easier to find unsweetened.

Beverages labeled "natural" are not guaranteed to be GE-free.[20]

Quick Hints – organic

Choose certified organic juices and sodas; avoid those containing corn syrup, aspartame, and other corn- or soy-derived ingredients

CHECKING OUT

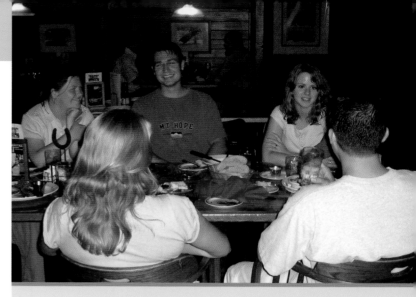

Thus ends our tour through the aisles of the supermarket. We've seen that avoiding GE foods is possible, as GE-free options abound in every corner of the grocery store. We hope you are now better equipped to go completely GE-free. Refer frequently to this guide; identifying GE-free options will become second nature. And remember, for more in-depth information, consult the shopping list in Appendix 1 for a comprehensive overview of popular brand products, and start voting out GE items with your food dollars!

WHEN EATING OUT: TIPS TO AVOID GE FOODS

1. Order organic meats, chicken, and sustainably raised fish which are presently not genetically engineered.

2. Avoid foods that contain large amounts of corn and soy, unless you are sure those ingredients are organic or certified GE-free.

3. Avoid foods cooked or fried in conventional corn, soybean, cottonseed, and canola oils. Choose foods cooked in pure olive, sesame, sunflower, safflower, almond, and peanut oils. Ask the restaurant staff to identify what kinds of oils are used in cooking.

4. Order foods that are made with dairy products that are organic or rbGH free.

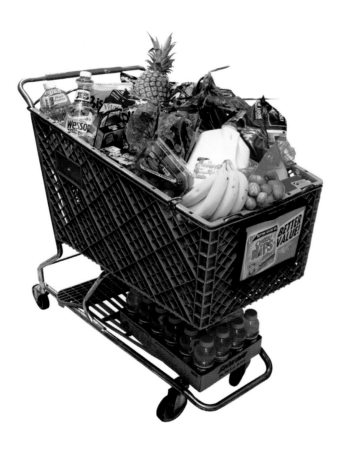

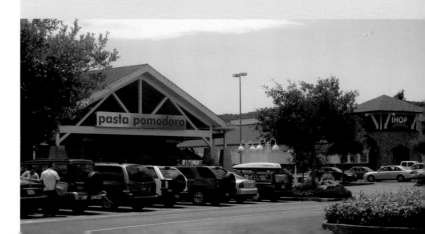

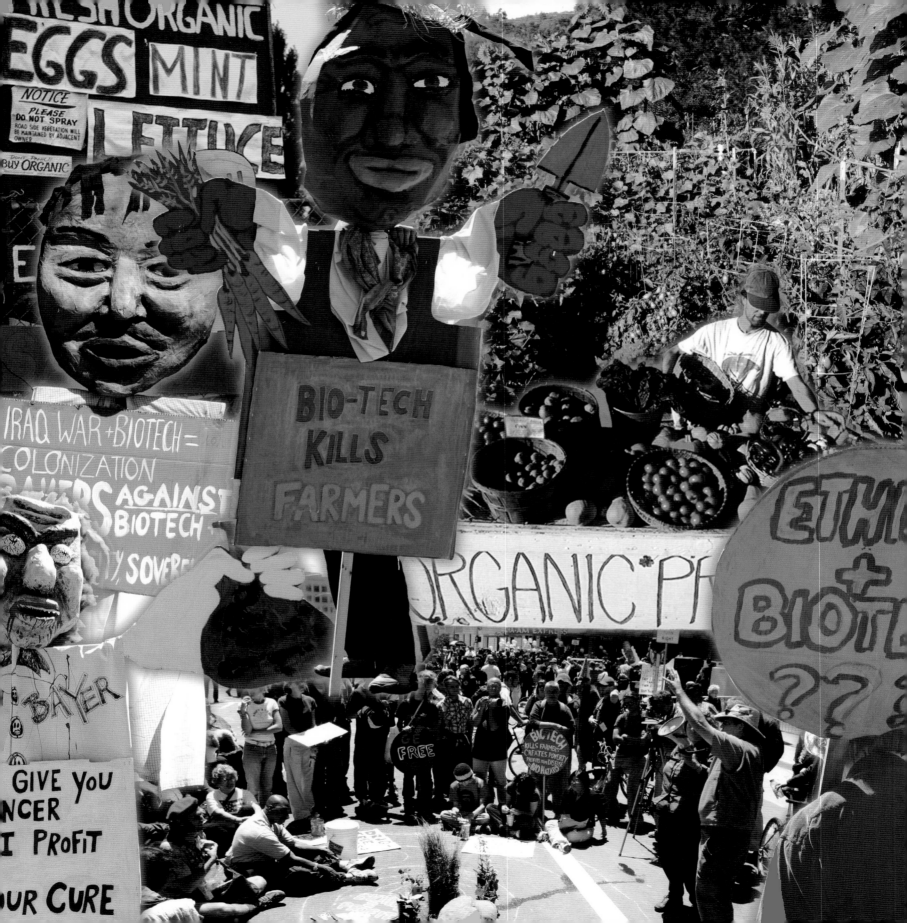

CHAPTER FIVE

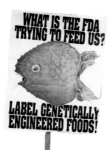

Choosing the Future of Food

an Activist speaks out

ELS COOPERRIDER was born in a small village in Holland. She immigrated to the U.S. with her family and came to Mendocino County when she was 16. Els received her bachelor's degree in botany from the University of California, Berkeley, and a master's degree in range science. With her husband and two sons, she owns and operates the first certified organic brewpub in the United States, Ukiah Brewing Co. & Restaurant.

ELS COOPERRIDER, OWNER AND OPERATOR OF UKIAH BREWING CO. & RESTAURANT, TELLS WHY SHE'S CONCERNED ABOUT GE FOODS.

I grew up in a Holland devastated by a world war and German occupation: everyone was struggling to get back on their feet, dealing with neighbors' lost families and concentration camp horror stories. The nonstop terror and violence around me taught me a great deal about injustice, and that burden established a strong personal value system. Also, my parents were members of the Dutch Resistance, hiding Jews and Allied airmen and fleeing resistance fighters. So when confronted with the choices between challenging something unjust and ignoring it, I could not help but stand up to the task.

After immigrating with my family to America, I received a bachelor's degree in botany from the University of California, Berkeley and a master's degree in Range Science. But wherever I went into the academic and science communities, I would often see greed or corruption—and I would confront it. After blowing the whistle on a contraband radioactive materials operation, I was fired. It became nearly impossible to get another job and to make ends meet.

With our two boys grown and on their own, my husband Allen and I came back to California to live in a small cabin in the woods in Mendocino County. The cabin had been in Allen's family and was situated along a creek, off the grid and without phone service. It was a few miles from Comptche, the nearest small town. But even in Mendocino, we kept fighting the good fight. I began involving myself in local politics and environmental matters and led an effort to ban roadside pesticide spraying in the county. We took on the Department of Transportation, and today Mendocino is the only county in California where both the county and state mow roadside weeds instead of killing them with toxic chemicals.

My son Bret, a brewer, wanted to join us in Mendocino and start his own brewery, so we helped raise investment funds with family, community, and small business loans. Together, the family started the Ukiah Brewing Company & Restaurant. I insisted that the beer and food we served there had to be organic (which hadn't been done before in the country)—for the environment and everything it entails, for the workers in the field, and for the people who eat and drink. I would not have been involved if our venture weren't going to be organic.

Today, we are the first certified-organic brewpub and the second certified-organic restaurant in the country. Our goal is to make a living, not a "killing." We want to provide good organic food at a reasonable, affordable price. We also talked about a place that would be a social center, but we didn't think it would actually turn out the way it has. It took about three years for it to become an unofficial town hall. Three vital community and food organizations were founded and grew at the brewery, along with the local alternative newspaper, *The Bullhorn*. I'm a co-founder of those groups, which includes the Mendocino Organic Network, a small group of volunteers offering certification services for independent, local, organic farmers. Our label, which we call Mendocino Renegade, stands for better standards and the support of local farmers. During a meeting of the Mendocino Organic Network, I suggested that we try to ban genetically modified organisms from the county.

Having studied biology for many years, I realized that GE researchers were picking apart the very essence of life and reorganizing it as if they were God. This was so preposterous that I couldn't just sit by and let it happen. It wasn't because I have a religious belief about it, but because I realized that organisms here for three million years must be created by nature over many millennia. Innumerable random mutations and natural selection gave us soybeans and corn. Now people have just decided to start playing with those genetics, adding genes from other species, which we would never see in nature. It's as if those millions of years of natural development were for naught. This is short-sighted thinking, and it's causing havoc—with much worse to come. We're already seeing widespread seed contamination, crop failures, infestations, and "super weeds," but we really haven't seen all the damage that these organisms can cause. I love my community; the potential negative consequences to it—and to our personal and collective health—affront our dignity. Polls show an overwhelming citizen demand that GMOs be at least labeled on our food, yet the biotech industry and the government refuse to comply with the public's wishes.

My training as a botanist led me to realize that genetic engineering of plants is a kind of ecological roulette, driven by money and greed, without consideration of the environmental, human health, or economic consequences. So I proposed that we write up an ordinance to ban GMO crops from our county, and then either ask the board of supervisors to enact it or we would collect signatures and put the initiative on the ballot. We knew very well that we could be taking on multinational corporations with countless billions of dollars at their disposal; however, we didn't know whether they would actually come into the county and try to stop us. They did.

Mendocino County voters defeated the world's largest producers of genetically engineered foods and seed, who pumped a record $621,000 in political spending into a county of 47,000 voters. Monsanto, DuPont, Dow Chemical, and a consortium of other biotech multinational corporations shattered spending records in our small agricultural county. They were no match for thousands of Mendocino County farmers, business owners, vintners, and families who joined the largest, most successful grassroots campaign the county has ever seen to fight the encroachment of genetically engineered crops. We're the first county in the U.S. to prohibit the growing of genetically engineered crops and animals—but we won't be the last. We proved that no amount of money can replace the love and commitment of people who care passionately about their community. This is a turning point in the corporate domination of the food system and a reclaiming of responsibility for agriculture at a local level.

They had the money, but we had the people.

The Voters Speak

In March 2004, voters in Mendocino County, CA passed a bill that bans the planting of GE crops in their county. Since that time, several other counties in California have brought this issue to their voters and/or county board of supervisors. Marin County passed a ballot initiative to ban the planting of GE crops, and the board of supervisors in Trinity County, CA passed a similar measure. Other counties including Sonoma, San Luis Obispo, and Butte also brought ballot initiatives to their voters, fought worthy battles, and educated tens of thousands of members of their communities about the potential hazards of GE crops. The biotech industry poured hundreds of thousands of dollars into fighting against these initiatives and, some believe, disseminating false or misleading information to the public leading to the defeat of these measures. Although these counties lost their ballot initiatives (most by slim margins), the educational and outreach efforts within the community proved to be a success.

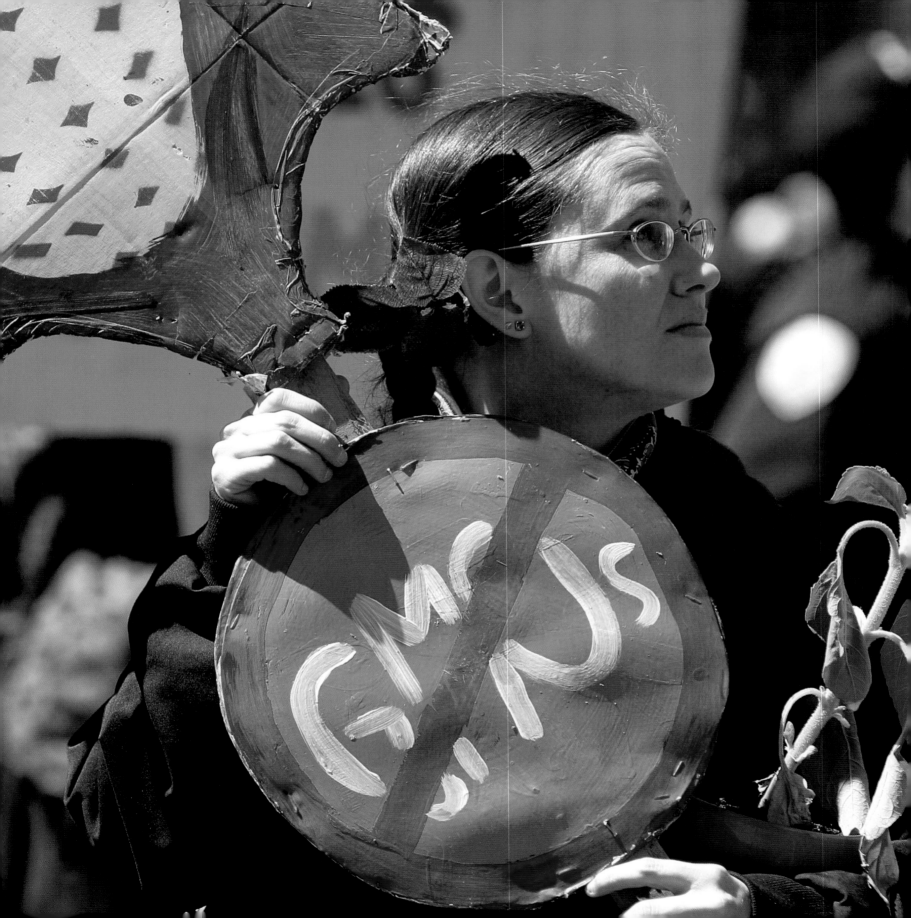

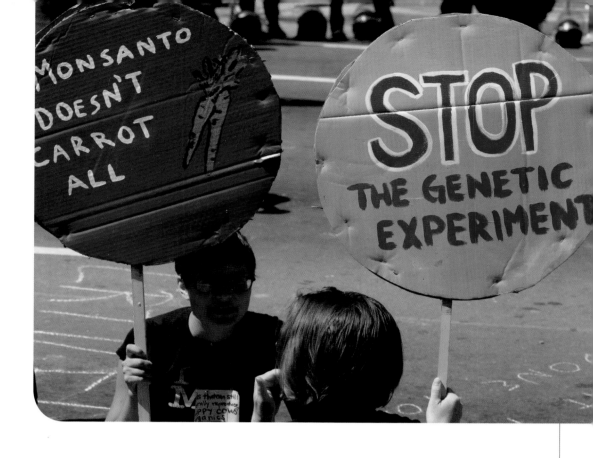

10 Ways to Get Involved!

We all have the right to choose the future of our food and we all have the power to make a difference. What can you do?

Lots! From cities and counties passing local measures restricting GE crops to two Alabama grandmothers distributing fliers on GE food in front of their local supermarket, people all over our nation and the world have taken action to stop the genetic engineering of our foods, our farms, and our futures. There is no limit to the ways in which we can put a stop to the genetic experiment with our food supply. In this chapter, we give you ten effective methods to become involved, and share some success stories of people around the country. Even if you choose only one of these actions, you can make a big difference.

"[There are] a multitude of purposes for which Earth Charter can be used [including]... citizen participation in environmental and educational programs...and even local campaigns against genetically modified organisms." [1]

—*Mikhail Gorbachev*
Former leader of the Soviet Union,
1990 Nobel Peace Prize Winner

1 SPREAD THE WORD!

Most people discuss current events with their friends and co-workers. Friends listen to and respect each other's opinions. If genetic engineering is important to you, talk to friends, family, and people in your community about it. Write one thing you will do to promote the mission of this book on the inside cover and pass the book along to a friend. Ask them to do the same.

Spreading the word is simple. Whenever you receive an e-mail on an issue or event you find important, forward it to a friend, or better yet, include ten friends. Start an online petition and ask your friends and family to sign it and circulate it. Many people e-mail news articles to their friends that address the issues they care about. These are all good ways to get people interested and involved. The greatest successes often come from simple actions that engage people on a personal level, not expensive advertising or celebrity endorsements.

SUCCESS STORY!

The People Take on The USDA: Protecting Organic Standards

In December 1997, under pressure from big agribusiness, the USDA suggested weakening the proposed organic standards by allowing genetic engineering, sewage sludge, and irradiation in organic food production. The USDA also refused to heed the recommendations or respect the authority of the National Organic Standards Board (NOSB), a citizen's board with the legal authority to provide recommendations to the USDA's Secretary of Agriculture. The largest and most negative public campaign in USDA history followed.

More than a quarter of a million people flooded the USDA with letters, e-mails, and phone calls in opposition of the agency's attempt to undermine organic farming. This unprecedented public outrage forced the USDA to reverse its position and declare that "the big three"—genetic engineering, sewage sludge, and irradiation—would not be in any re-proposed organic rulings. They also announced that any future organic standards proposal would respect the authority of the NOSB.

These public comments came from many places. Citizens signed petitions and forwarded e-mails among friends and family, shoppers brought postcards to workplaces and to supermarkets, and people spread the word by talking to each other about protecting the integrity of organic food and farming. Though advocates of organic farming standards continue to fight the industry's recurring attempts to erode these important guidelines, the public campaign remains a landmark victory for organic farmers and the vast number of people who took action to support them.

Take Action Now!

⇨ To start a free online petition, visit www.thepetitionsite.com

⇨ Spruce up your e-mails. Make them more entertaining by employing free e-cards and e-postcards. Find them through a simple Web search or personalize your message with your own digital photos.

⇨ Many online news providers provide an "e-mail this article" link where you can send information to your friends for free. Most provide space for you to enter a short personal message as well.

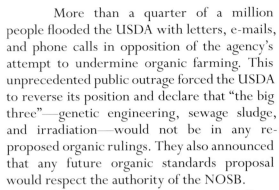

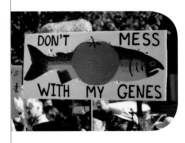

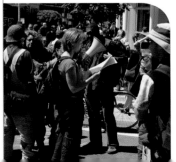

2 B.Y.O.B.—BEGIN IN YOUR OWN BACKYARD

You've often heard it said that change begins at home. There are a number of things you can do in your community to make a difference. One is growing organic food. Even if you just grow potted herbs on your deck, it's a great way to rekindle your connection to the food you eat and the land that produces it. If you can't garden at home, find a local community garden or start one with friends and neighbors. Community gardens allow you to grow your own organic produce while connecting you to others who share your interest in this issue.

There are many fun and creative ways you can get your community involved. Nothing brings people together better than good food, so invite your friends and neighbors to an organic potluck dinner or brunch. Discuss the reasons this issue is so important to you and find out why it's important to your friends. One local activist created a pin-the-gene-on-the-tomato game to discuss the issue. Be entertaining, be inspiring, be informative and have fun!

(See "Resources for Gardening" on page 102 for info on where to buy organic seeds and starts, information on community gardens, alternatives to chemicals in the garden, and ideas for gatherings, events, and community organizing.)

SUCCESS STORY!

Alice Waters and the Edible Schoolyard

Alice Waters is an award-winning chef, author and food activist in Berkeley, California. You probably know her best as the founder of Chez Panisse restaurant, which she opened in the 1970s. But Alice hasn't stopped there. She brought her creative genius and her love of lo-cal, organic foods to the students of Berkeley's Martin Luther King, Jr. Middle School. Waters gathered parents and community members there to start the Edible Schoolyard.

She described the Edible Schoolyard project in a chapter she wrote for *Fatal Harvest: The Tragedy of Industrial Agriculture:*

For years, whenever I drove by the school, I was struck by how rundown the schoolyard looked, and I thought, what a great garden this would make. And what a great thing it would be if the students not only got to plan, plant, and cultivate the garden, but if they actually got to use that food to cook school lunches for themselves. To my delight, the principal of the school thought this was a good idea, too.

The kids are very receptive. Now at King School, they are getting boxes of produce from a community supported agriculture farm—each class receives a box every week. One of the teachers was telling us at a garden design meeting for the schoolyard about how the kids in her class washed and trimmed and cut up the ingredients and made a big salad. "Now wait," she said. "Before we start eating, let's stop and think about the person who tilled the ground and planted the seeds and harvested the vegetables. And then we chopped up the vegetables and put them in this bowl and made this big salad..."—and the kids stood up at their desks and gave the salad a huge standing ovation.

Take Action Now!

⇨ For more information on the Edible School yard, including tips on starting an organic "edible schoolyard" project in your own community and links to organizations that can help, visit www.edibleschoolyard.org/homepage.html

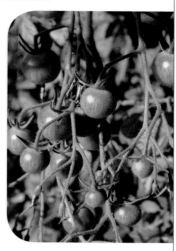

FACT

Cropland dedicated to organic agriculture more than doubled from 1992 to 1997 and doubled again between 1997 and 2003.

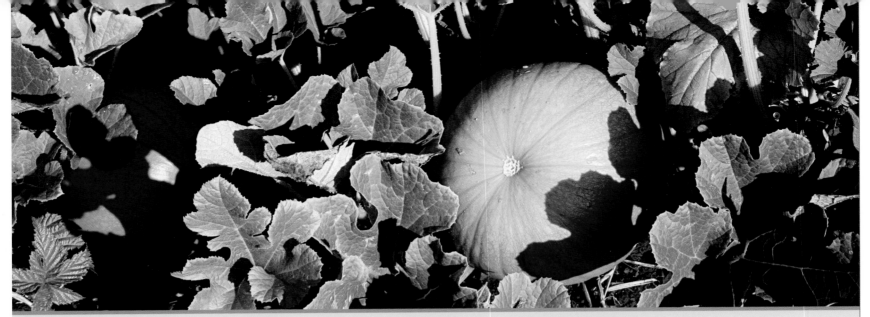

RESOURCES FOR GARDENING

Non-GE and Organic Seeds

FEDCO Seeds
Waterville, Maine
A cooperative seed and garden supply company.
www.fedcoseeds.com

Heirloom Seeds,
West Elizabeth, Pennsylvania
All seeds untreated, non-hybrid.
www.heirloomseeds.com

Golden Harvest Organics LLC
Fort Collins, Colorado
Non-GMO, organic heirloom tomato seeds.
www.ghorganics.com

Organic Seed Alliance
Port Townsend, Washington
Collaborative education and research programs with organic farmers and other seed professionals.
www.seedalliance.org

Peaceful Valley Farm Supply
Grass Valley, California
Huge seed assortment, organic fertilizers.
www.groworganic.com

Non-toxic Alternatives to Pesticides in Your Garden

There are several great resources to check out to learn how to garden organically and how to deal with pest problems without the use of chemical pesticides:

Pesticide Action Network North America (PANNA)
Offers a "pesticide advisor" with many good tips.
www.panna.org/resources/advisor.dv.html

Northwest Coalition for Alternatives to Pesticides
Offers a "Healthier Homes and Gardens" program, with free monthly garden tips and more.
www.pesticide.org/HHG.html

Beyond Pesticides
Lots of good information on common garden pests and how to control them.
www.beyondpesticides.org
www.groworganic.com

Community Gardens

The American Community Garden Association
ACGA has a wealth of resources to help you find, join or even start your own community garden.

For a list of community gardens by state, see www.communitygarden.org/links.php#Gardens

For tips on how to start a community garden, visit www.communitygarden.org/links.php#Generalcg

For great tips on urban and rooftop gardening, visit City Farmer at
www.cityfarmer.org/rooftop59.html

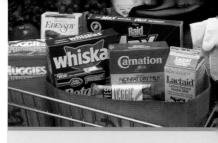

3 USE YOUR PERSONAL BUYING POWER

It's no wonder cropland dedicated to organic agriculture more than doubled from 1992 to 1997 and doubled again between 1997 and 2003.[3] Organic food sales are advancing by 20 percent every year, compared to the 2- to 5-percent growth of the food industry as a whole.[4] Everything from organic cotton clothing to salad dressings and herbal supplements is widely available in neighborhood shops and large grocery chains. Many supermarket chains even produce their own certified-organic store-brand products now because of high consumer demand.

Remember that "certified organic" means it's NOT genetically engineered. Federal organic standards don't allow the use of genetically modified seed.[5] Buying certified, 100 percent organic products is the one sure way to avoid unlabeled genetically engineered ingredients.

Also, steer clear of GE ingredients by selecting whole foods, including unprocessed fruits, vegetables, grains, beans, nuts, and seeds, as much as possible. The power of consumers' dollars can serve as votes against genetic engineering.

SUCCESS STORY!

Wielding Consumer Power: The Tillamook Story

The Tillamook County Creamery Association, the nation's second largest cheese-maker, announced in February 2005 it had asked all of its 147 member farmers to halt the use of recombinant bovine growth hormone (rBGH, sometimes also called rBST), despite increasing pressure from Monsanto to overturn that decision.

Tillamook told the *Associated Press* that shoppers influenced the decision to ban the hormone. "Consumers of Tillamook dairy products expect Tillamook to do the right thing," they said. "They're asking us to remove the recombinant bovine hormone from our product and we're just responding to that."

The dairy cooperative said that Monsanto sent an attorney from its Washington, D.C. law firm to meet with more than a dozen co-op members. But in an incredible display of consumer activism, more than 6,500 people contacted Tillamook by phone, e-mail, fax, or letter. More than 98 percent of the comments supported the dairy's decision to go rBGH-free. Consumer activism works.

Take Action Now!

⇨ For more information on the effort to make Tillamook rbGH-free, visit www.oregonpsr.org/programs/campaign SafeFood.html

4 THINK GLOBALLY, BUY LOCALLY: FARM-FRESH FOODS

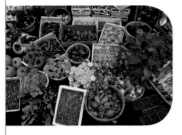

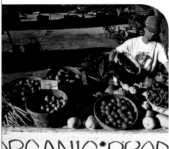

"Free people with free information are saying no to genetically engineered food for both ecological and health reasons. However, genetic engineering is being imposed on the world by a handful of global corporations with the backing of one powerful government."[7]

—*Dr. Vandana Shiva*
Physicist, activist, and author

Alarmed by industrial agriculture's interference in the food chain? It's easy to meet local growers who cherish the land. Look for farmers' markets where growers sell directly to the public. As the number of farmers' markets has surged to 3,000, nearly doubling in the past decade, one is sure to be nearby.

Sign up with a Community Supported Agriculture (CSA) farm to feel secure about where the food you're eating comes from. As part of an annual subscription, households receive a basket of fresh, locally grown produce throughout the growing season. There are more than 1,000 Community Supported Agriculture farms coast to coast.

Does Your Food Travel More than You Do?

Our food travels an average of 1,300 miles from the farm to the dinner table.[8] Subsequently, consumers get farther away from their food sources while farmers command lower prices for their products. For every dollar a consumer spends on food, farmers receive ten cents or less. Just a few decades ago, farmers earned up to seventy cents.[9] More and more of our food dollars go to the middlemen for processing, packaging, storing, and shipping, and the people who actually grow it receive increasingly less. But the good news is that more and more consumers want to buy and eat locally grown foods. A 2004 national poll conducted by Roper Public Affairs for Organic Valley Family of Farms[10] showed that 73 percent of Americans want to know whether or not their food is grown or produced locally and regionally.

Take Action Now!

⇨ For information on how to get involved in or start a "Buy Local" campaign in your area, visit www.foodroutes.org.

Waiter, There's a Fly Gene in My Soup!

Restaurants are searching out ways to buy local, sustainable agriculture too. Many chefs take pride in fresh, local, often organic ingredients and humanely raised meat and dairy. Menus will usually highlight this approach. If you don't see it, ask. Remember, forty-two cents of every family food dollar is spent on meals away from home (see "Vote with Your Food Dollars", p.103). Where do you want to spend yours?

Take Action Now!

⇨ For more information on what chefs and restaurants are doing, including a Restaurant Guide, visit the Chef's Collaborative at www.chefscollaborative.org
⇨ Find a farmers' market or a Community Supported Agriculture (CSA) farm at www.ams.usda.gov/farmersmarkets www.localharvest.com

5 MAY I SPEAK TO THE MANAGER? TALKING TO PEOPLE WITH PURCHASING POWER

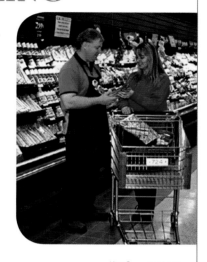

Supermarket activism was extremely important and effective in forcing genetically engineered food off the shelves throughout Europe. In the U.S., we are starting to see some of those same results. Whole Foods and Wild Oats, two national supermarket chains, have pledged to sell exclusively non-GE ingredients in their store-brand products. Trader Joe's, after about a year of grassroots consumer campaigning, pledged to source non-GE ingredients for all of their store-brand products. Texas-based supermarket HEB recently introduced their line of labeled, GE-free, store-brand items after years of consumer pressure. These victories prove that supermarkets can make this change. Perhaps more importantly, this triumph shows that if we work together, change will happen.

Take Back the Aisles!

Supermarkets are important because:

- They control a large amount of food production through their store-brand products.
- They are the part of the food industry that has the most exposure and most immediate accountability to the public.
- They must answer to their customers and the public. The supermarket industry is highly competitive and the profit margins are relatively slim, so what you purchase—or more importantly, don't purchase—has an impact.

Speaking to supermarket store managers is easier than you think. When you do, let them know your concerns about GE foods. Ask them to remove GE ingredients from their store-brand products, as other supermarkets have already done. Request more organic and non-GE alternatives for the products you usually purchase. If the manager isn't available, fill out a customer card with your concerns.

Take Action Now!

⇨ Supermarkets across the country are being urged to go GE-free. To get involved where you live, download the Supermarket Activist Kit or, find more information on supermarket campaigns, visit www.truefoodnow.org/supermarkets. (Check the "Resources" section for a sample letter to supermarket managers.)

Who Else Needs to Know How You Feel?

The food companies that use genetically engineered ingredients need to know! Some major companies, including Gerber and Frito-Lay, have already pledged not to use these ingredients in some of their products. Consumer activism persuaded Whole Foods, Wild Oats, and Trader Joe's to remove GE ingredients from their store-brand products. Several large dairy companies, including Tillamook, have asked their dairy farmers to banish Monsanto's rBGH in response to customer demands. Even McDonald's, out of fear that consumers would not buy their french fries, pledged to avoid GE potatoes. You have tremendous power as

"The 2001 announcement by Trader Joe's marks the first time a mainstream grocery chain has dropped GE ingredients in response to consumer demand. By responding to its customers, Trader Joe's has set an industry standard and has helped put other mainstream retailers on notice —they can't say "we can't make GE free products in the U.S." anymore."

—*Heather Whitehead*
True Food Network Director

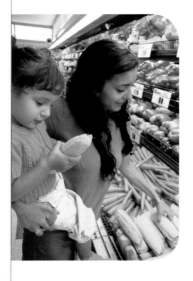

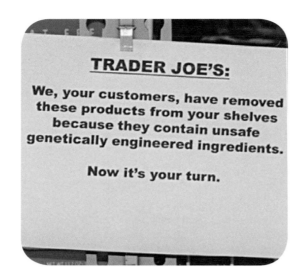

TRADER JOE'S:

We, your customers, have removed these products from your shelves because they contain unsafe genetically engineered ingredients.

Now it's your turn.

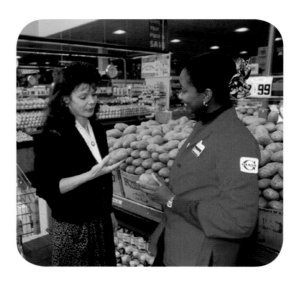

"We are not yet in a position to assess the biological disturbance that could result from indiscriminate genetic manipulation and from the unscrupulous development of new forms of plant and animal life....It is evident that in any area as delicate as this, indifference to fundamental ethical norms, or their rejection, would lead humankind to the very threshold of self-destruction."[11]

—Pope John Paul II

a consumer—use it! (Check the Appendix for addresses of America's largest food companies.)

SUCCESS STORY!

Texas Grocer Feels the Heat

At the end of April 2001, Texas consumers concerned about GMO contamination exercised their right to choose and launched a write-in campaign to HEB, a major Texas grocery chain. HEB is a $10.5 billion family-owned Texas business, the largest privately held company in the state, with more than 300 stores and 50,000 employees.

Within a few weeks, HEB offered to meet with the Texas-based group, Say No to GMOs! Three high-level HEB representatives met with seven concerned Texas consumers for more than two hours. This was the first step toward finding solutions to the lack of consumer choice in the marketplace.

A growing coalition of organizations and consumer advocates made repeated re-

quests for a follow-up meeting with HEB. HEB was at first unresponsive, but after the Texas consumer activists added pressure with a rally at the company's corporate offices, HEB granted the group a second meeting.

In 2005, HEB announced new Central Market Organic and Central Market All-Natural product lines. While other supermarkets manufacture store-brand products that are GMO-free, HEB is the first to actually label their non-GMO products: "This product was made from ingredients that were not grown from genetically modified seed." While this is a significant victory and a great first step by the company, Say No to GMOs! and other Texas consumers are pushing HEB to expand their non-GE options to all of their store-brand products.

Take Action Now!

⇨ For more information on Say No to GMOs! and the HEB campaign in Texas, visit www.saynotogmos.org

6 SHOP WITH SHARED VALUES: CHANGING THE BUYING POWER IN YOUR COMMUNITY

We can encourage the purchasing of fresh, local and organic foods. School lunch programs across the country are buying more local, organic produce; workplace cafeterias are sourcing more organic foods; hospitals are bringing farmers' markets to their parking lots; and city councils are asking that local, organic foods be a part of city events. Even some college agriculture programs are making their campus farms and gardens all organic. The following are some examples of success stories according to the Organic Trade Association:[12]

SUCCESS STORY!

Kaiser Permanente, one of the largest health care providers in the West, welcomes farmers' markets at some of its medical centers. Since May 2003, the weekly farmers' market at Kaiser's Oakland hospital draws as many as 1,000 employees, physicians, patients, and neighbors. Kaiser's San Francisco center has also started a farmers' market and Kaiser's Hawaii unit has launched similar venues. In 2004, Kaiser opened an organic farm stand at its Richmond, California medical center, where low-income neighborhood residents can buy hard-to-find fresh produce. Farmers' markets have also started up at Kaiser's Santa Theresa and Santa Clara medical centers.

Olympia, Washington grade schools offer organic salad bars to their students. Lincoln Elementary in Olympia cut its lunch costs by two cents a meal even though it offers a full organic menu.

Seattle's school district recently adopted a policy to ban foods high in sugar and fat. The district encourages serving organic food in school cafeterias whenever feasible. The school board policy is available at www.seattleschools.org/area/policies/index.dxml

Yale University has expanded its sustainable-food menu to include organic entrees due to demand. Yale also extended organic-meal service from one dining hall to ten.

Delaware Valley College is seeking organic certification from Pennsylvania Certified Organic for its two-acre plot devoted to growing blueberries, snap beans, and corn.

Take Action Now!

⇨ For information on bringing fresh, local, and organic foods into your schools and institutions, visit the Community Food Security Coalition at www.foodsecurity.org

⇨ To join or start a GM-Free School project, check out the Institute for Responsible Technology's GM-Free Schools Campaign at www.gmfreeschools.org. They offer videos, audio CDs, and many other resources to help you work with your local school district as well as rallying organizational support and setting up Web hosting for your local efforts.

⇨ For tips on working with your schools, see www.theorganicreport.com. Click on the O'Kid link, scroll to the bottom of the page and select the article, "Organic Foods in Schools—Eleven Tips for Change."

⇨ Visit the Organic Trade Association at www.ota.com

FACT

There are more than 1,000 Community Supported Agriculture (CSA) farms coast to coast.

7 GET ORGANIZED: JOIN OR START A LOCAL GROUP

Joining a local group is a great way to get active in changing the future of food and to meet like-minded people in your community. Try organic gardening clubs and local chapters of larger, sustainable-agriculture groups to get started. Many national organizations offer resources and assistance to local groups of activists working on similar campaigns. Contact these organizations and ask about programs that assist local, grass-roots efforts. (See Appendix 3A for a list of sustainable agriculture organizations)

If you can't find a group in your community, start your own

As famed sociologist Margaret Mead once said: "Never doubt that the actions of a few committed citizens can change the world. Indeed, it's the only thing that ever has." The Sierra Club, an environmental watchdog group, is a shining example of what happens when people join together. A handful of citizens, including conservationist John Muir, founded the group in 1892. Today, the Sierra Club, 700,000 members strong, is the nation's largest grassroots environmental organization.

Amnesty International (AI) started forty years ago with one man's inspiring article in the British newspaper, *The Observer*; AI now has nearly two million members around the world. Thousands of small grassroots groups dot the country today—groups of neighbors, friends, and co-workers organizing together to create change and raise awareness. They're making a big difference. (Check the Appendix for information and help on starting a local group, recruiting volunteers, planning and running a community meeting, and other tips.)

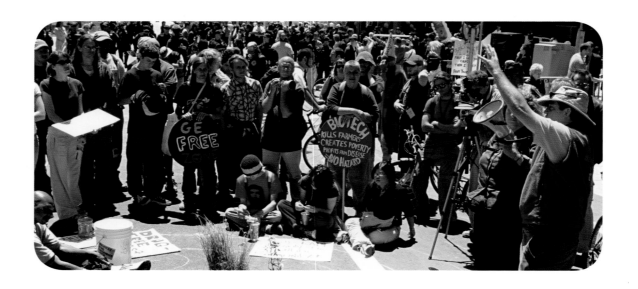

GMO-free Hawaii

In 2002, organic farmers, parents, teachers and concerned citizens learned that Hawaii was the genetic engineering capital of the world. The state permitted more field trial sites than any other place on the planet. Very quickly, a grassroots movement developed. The group—comprised of GMO-Free Maui; GMO-Free O'ahu, GMO-Free Kaua'i, and on the Big Island, Hawai'i GEAN (HIGEAN)—is working to protect Hawaii's environment and people from the risks of genetically modified crops. They joined forces and created a statewide coalition, GMO-Free Hawai'i. Today, 5,000 state residents have signed on in support of the coalition's campaign. The group has worked with state agriculture boards, farmers associations, individual farmers, and farmers' markets. In 2005, GMO-Free Kaua'i successfully developed the first GMO-FREE farmers' market in the Aloha State. Meanwhile another coalition member, HIGEAN, has hosted three annual seed exchanges and seed-saving workshops attended by 200 farmers each year.

Though GMO-Free Hawai'i has just a few organizers on each island, their accomplishments are huge. In the past three years, these groups have had a major impact on several campaigns:

•GMO Coffee: The coalition saw three major resolutions passed by the Kona Coffee Council, the Kona Farm Bureau and the Hawaii County Council. The group also helped broker an agreement that effectively halted the development and growing of GMO coffee in the state.

•GMO Papaya: GMO-Free Hawai'i began conducting contamination tests for concerned community farmers and soon discovered alarming levels of contamination on the major islands. The announcement of their test results received extensive coverage in the state, the *New York Times*, *USA Today,* and publications reaching millions of readers across the world.

•GMO Taro: In 2005, some of their collaborative partners negotiated an agreement with the University f Hawai'i to stop all GMO research on Hawaiian varieties of taro, an important native food plant.

•Legal Action: GMO-Free Hawai'i worked with the Center for Food Safety and Earthjustice, a nonprofit law firm, on a lawsuit to force the U.S. Department of Agriculture to disclose field trial sites for GMO biopharmaceutical crops in Hawaii. Since the filing of the lawsuit, all biopharmaceutical field trials have pulled out of the state.

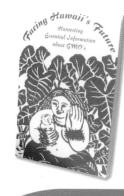

Facing Hawaii's Future: Harvesting Essential Information about GMOs

Hawaii's priceless living treasure of complex ecosystems is under siege today. This island state has produced a bounty of unique produce (papaya, coffee, macadamia nuts, and sugar cane, to name a few) for the rest of the continental United States, so why would large food corporations want a hand in changing the face of farming in Hawaii? As it turns out, Hawaii is considered to be a "ground zero" for the open field testing of genetically modified organisms. Hawai'i SEED, also known as GMO-Free Hawai'i, created in reaction to information about the effects of genetically modified organisms and the reason behind worldwide resistance to this agricultural technology. In addition to defining what exactly is a GMO, this booklet provides solutions on how to become a more informed consumer and resources for further action. *Facing Hawaii's Future* is beautifully illustrated by artist Mayumi Oda.

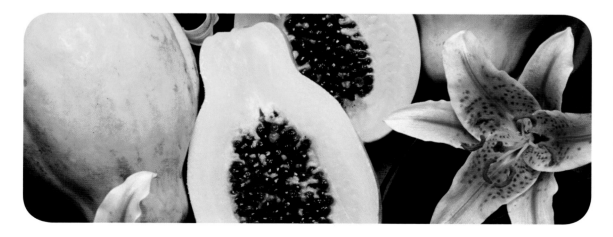

8 Don't Like the News? Go Out and Make Your Own: Using Your Local Media

FACT

For every dollar a consumer spends on food, farmers receive ten cents or less. Just a few decades ago, farmers earned up to seventy cents.

More and more people are turning to alternative media outlets and the Internet to get news outside of the mainstream and views from news sources abroad. Many have also decided to make their own media. Concerned citizens are spreading the word through websites, flash animation projects, submissions to online organizations such as the Independent Media Center, and documentary films on subjects they care about and feel are under-represented in the mainstream press.

Of course, not everyone can make a documentary. Nevertheless, you do have plenty of other opportunities to use local media or make your own. Most newspapers have opinion or editorial sections you may be able to contribute to and almost all papers print letters to the editor. These are easy, no-cost ways to convey your views in the press.

If you are running or starting a local campaign, chances are the media will be in-terested in the story. Never think they won't care. Always contact them when you have a large event planned—a rally, a supermarket tour, or a school board meeting about the lunch program, for example. Community members want to know what's happening and often, the local press relies on people like you—the organizers or attendees of the event—to let them know the details and its importance to citizens.

Take Action Now!

⇨ For information on working with the media and a community media guide including sample press advisories and releases, see Appendix 2.

⇨ Alternative media sites:
Independent Media Center:
www.indymedia.org
Guerilla News Network: www.gnn.tv
Free Press: www.freepress.net

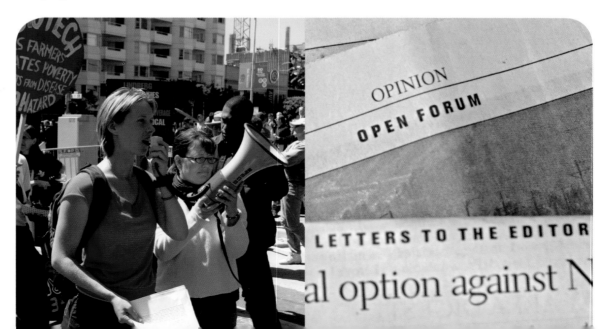

The Future of Food

Deborah Koons Garcia has been a filmmaker for over thirty years and she operates her own film company, Lily Films. She has always been conscious of her food choices and the impact she has when making them. While mulling over a documentary on pesticide issues, she stumbled onto something even larger. Discussing her film *The Future of Food*, Garcia told the *San Francisco Chronicle*:[14]

"It became clear that GMOs are really a much bigger issue ... Someone needed to make this film because if this technology isn't challenged and if this corporatization of our whole food system isn't stopped, at some point it will be too late.

"I want people to watch the film and say, 'We have to stop this.'"

Long gone are the days when Garcia believed, "We could have our healthy foods over here, and they could have their food over there. You do your thing and I do mine." With genetic engineering, she says, "You can't drop out anymore—it'll come and get us."

After three years of filming across the U.S., Canada, and Mexico, thousands of people have seen *The Future of Food*. Local groups nationwide are using the film to get their communities involved in the movement against GE foods. And it's working. The first success came when California's Mendocino County passed the first-ever county-level ban on the growing of GE crops in 2004. *The Future of Food* was shown several times there as a work-in-progress.

Take Action Now!

⇨ For more information on *The Future of Food* or to order your own copy, visit www.thefutureoffood.com

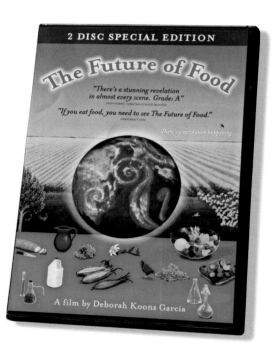

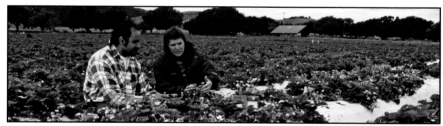

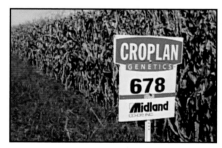

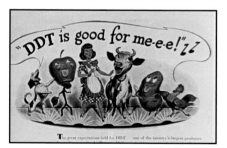

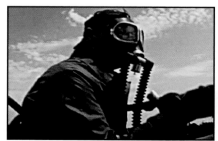

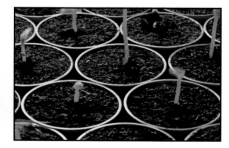

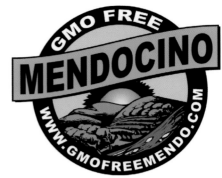

9 FOOD AND POLITICS: EMPOWERING DEMOCRACY

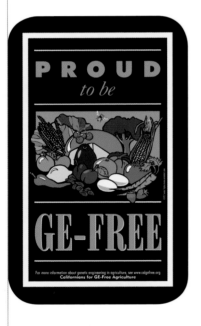

Build on your personal and community commitments to support a safe and sustainable food chain. Take it nationwide. Because so much of our food crosses state and national borders to get to the grocery store, the federal government plays an important role in forming these policies.

That means your representatives and senators need to hear what you think about genetic engineering. You can be sure the biotech industry is lobbying hard and making its case, and Capitol Hill deserves to hear both sides. Reasoned letters from constituents like you can be very persuasive. Look at the victories:

The Center for Food Safety and other nonprofit, public-interest organizations frequently ask the public to challenge weak and faulty regulatory policies at the federal level. In 2000, for example, the Center for Food Safety spearheaded an unprecedented coalition of science, consumer, environmental, and farm, organizations to petition the U.S. Food and Drug Administration to develop mandatory labeling guidelines and a thorough testing regime for genetically modified food. This petition impelled the agency to create an official rulemaking docket, which allowed the public to write in and support the initiative. More than 600,000 Americans wrote to the FDA to support the petition.

Write Your Congressperson

Look up your state and federal representatives' addresses at www.congress.org. Send letters to state and national legislators expressing your concerns about GE foods. Ask them to support mandatory labeling for genetically engineered foods. Encourage them to introduce or foster liability legislation that puts the responsibility of GE crop contamination not on farmers, but on producers such as Monsanto. Tell them we need mandatory, independent, long-term studies on the environmental and human health impacts of genetic engineering in food and agriculture.

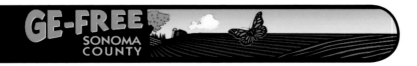

Democracy in Action

In March 2004, California's Mendocino County became the first in the country to pass a ballot initiative banning the cultivation of genetically engineered plants and animals countywide. Since then, Trinity, Marin, and Santa Cruz counties have passed similar laws in California.

In recent years, volunteers in Vermont and Massachusetts have succeeded in passing town-level legislation. Some call for proper labeling and appropriate regulation of genetically altered foods and crops; others have requested a moratorium on the local cultivation of genetically engineered crops.

Legislators have leaned toward full disclosure too. In the summer of 2004, after years of careful groundwork, activists in Vermont witnessed their state legislature pass the first law in the U.S. requiring the labeling of all genetically modified seeds statewide. This milestone represents a major step toward protecting growers, human health, and the environment. In Alaska, state law requires the labeling of any GE fish or fish product that is commercialized and sold in the state.

Take Action Now!

⇨ For more information on town and county resolutions and initiatives, visit www.gmofreemendo.org or www.gefreesonoma.org

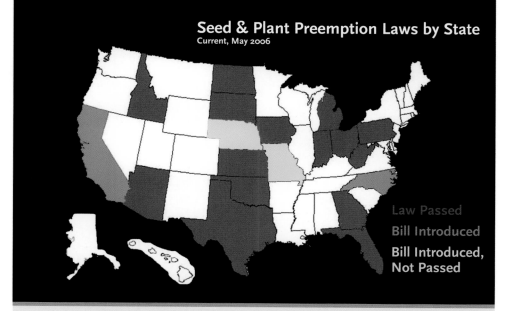

Seed & Plant Preemption Laws by State
Current, May 2006

Law Passed
Bill Introduced
Bill Introduced, Not Passed

LOCAL INITIATIVES THREATENED BY STATE LEGISLATION

In late 2004, the American Farm Bureau Federation, in association with the biotech industry, attempted to push legislation that would ban several state legislatures from passing local laws to regulate GE food. If enacted, the bills would effectively prohibit local governments and communities from enacting policies, ordinances and initiatives related to seeds and plants—including genetically engineered ones. These "Monsanto Laws" are a slap in the face of democracy.

By early 2006, this "preemption" legislation had already passed in fourteen states and was pending in four others, including California—the nation's largest agricultural state and the first to pass county-level restrictions on the growing of GE crops. Knowing where your state stands on this type of legislation is important. States passing or introducing preemption laws will take away local control and make any previous restrictions relating to GE seed or crop production unenforceable—even those passed by local voters.

Take Action Now!

⇨ Find out where your state stands by checking the Environmental Commons preemption tracker at www.environmentalcommons.org/gmo-tracker.html
⇨ Download your preemption toolkit and learn what you can do to stop this legislation in your state at www.centerforfoodsafety.org/preemptiontoolkit.cfm
⇨ For more information on GE-Free zones, visit Californians for GE Free Agriculture at www.calgefree.org and The Organic Consumers Association's BioDemocracy Alliance at www.organicconsumers.org/ge-free.htm

10 STAY INFORMED, STAY INVOLVED. JOIN THE CENTER FOR FOOD SAFETY'S TRUE FOOD NETWORK

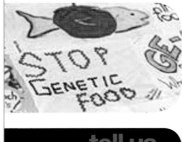

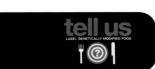

More than 30,000 True Food Network members have joined together to take collective action to stop the genetic experiment with our food and agriculture. True Food Network (TFN) members have worked on supermarket campaigns, local and state ballot initiatives and resolutions, petition drives, school lunch programs, and much more. TFN brings you news, campaign updates and easy ways you can make a difference and stand up for true food.

The True Food Network started in 2000 with 6,000 members; today, the network is more than 30,000 members strong. Together, TFN members have shared many successes:

• 2001: In less than a year, pressure from the TFN and allied grassroots groups brought Trader Joe's supermarkets to an agreement to remove all GE ingredients from their store-brand products.

• 2002: More than 300 events at supermarkets across the country and a network of TFN members helped bring national attention to the problems of GE food. More than 200 media stories nationwide focused on Local Supermarket Campaigns and the True Food Network.

• 2003-2004: True Food Network members played a critical role in the victory to stop the introduction of Monsanto's GE Roundup Ready wheat.

Sowing the Seeds of Change

Everybody's voice counts. Make sure yours is heard. Use your shopping dollars to vote against genetically engineered foods. Explore all the ways you can support the alternative—sustainable local agriculture that protects the land and our food chain. Join the Center for Food Safety's True Food Network to connect with thousands of citizens across the country concerned about genetic engineering.

Remember—genetic engineering is bringing radical, untested changes to our food supply. You have the right to know about the secret ingredients in what you eat. We all have the power to make a difference—and we all have the right to decide the future of food. Want to know more? Visit us online at www.centerforfoodsafety.org.

Take Action Now!

⇨ Join the True Food Network today by visiting www.truefoodnow.org or www.centerforfoodsafety.org.

Success Story!

Farmers Say No to Genetically Engineered Flax

Flaxseed has been getting more and more attention lately because it's an excellent source of Omega 3 essential fatty acids and other vitamins and minerals. So red flags went up in 2005, when the biotech start-up company Agragen announced its plan to grow trial plantings of GE flax in North Dakota. The flax was genetically engineered to produce albumin, a protein in human blood.[15] North Dakota grows more than 90 percent of the U.S. flax crop, so it didn't take long for flax farmers to speak up in defense of their products and their livelihoods. AmeriFlax, a branch of the North Dakota Oilseed Council, stated that "the risk of adulteration from genetic material not approved for food and feed entering the food chain is unacceptable..." Ernie Hoffert, the group's secretary-treasurer, summed up the objections of flax farmers when he stated, "Are we going to risk our new and emerging markets for flax on something that hasn't even been licensed yet? This is absurd."[16] He concluded, "There's nothing to gain and everything to lose."[17] Though Agragen has not publicly disavowed its plans for biopharm flax, the company has been conspicuously absent since the scuffle. Consumers have AmeriFlax to thank for defending flax products from possible contamination from the experimental genetically engineered variety.

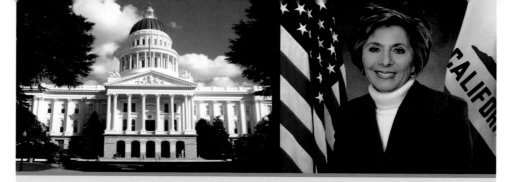

A LEGISLATOR SPEAKS OUT: BARBARA BOXER ON LABELING OF GE FOODS

If the United States required labeling of GE foods as European countries do, we wouldn't need this shopping guide. As early as 2000, U.S. Senator Barbara Boxer (D-CA) introduced a bill that would require the mandatory labeling of GE foods, asserting consumers' rights to know whether or not their food is genetically engineered. Yet Congress failed to act on this crucial legislation. The fight to require labeling continues and you can help. Meanwhile, the following letter, which Senator Boxer wrote not long before introducing her bill, provides much food for thought:[18]

February 8, 2000

Recent polls have demonstrated that Americans want to know if they are eating genetically engineered food. A January 1999 Time *magazine poll revealed that 81 percent of respondents wanted genetically engineered food to be labeled. A January 2000 MSNBC poll showed identical results...*

Given the rapid expansion of this largely untested technology, we should provide consumers with the right to know whether they are eating genetically engineered food. Congress has already provided consumers similar rights by requiring the labeling of foods containing artificial colors and flavors, chemical preservatives, and artificial sweeteners.

Labeling genetically engineered food would not be unprecedented for the U.S. In fact, as part of a recent 131-nation agreement to regulate trade in genetically engineered crops, the U.S. agreed to label its international shipments of seeds, grains, and plants that may contain genetically engineered material. If we can provide this information to our trading partners, shouldn't we make similar information available to American consumers?

Sincerely,
Barbara Boxer

GENETICALLY MODIFIED (GM) CROPS AND FOODS

WORLDWIDE REGULATION, PROHIBITION, AND PRODUCTION

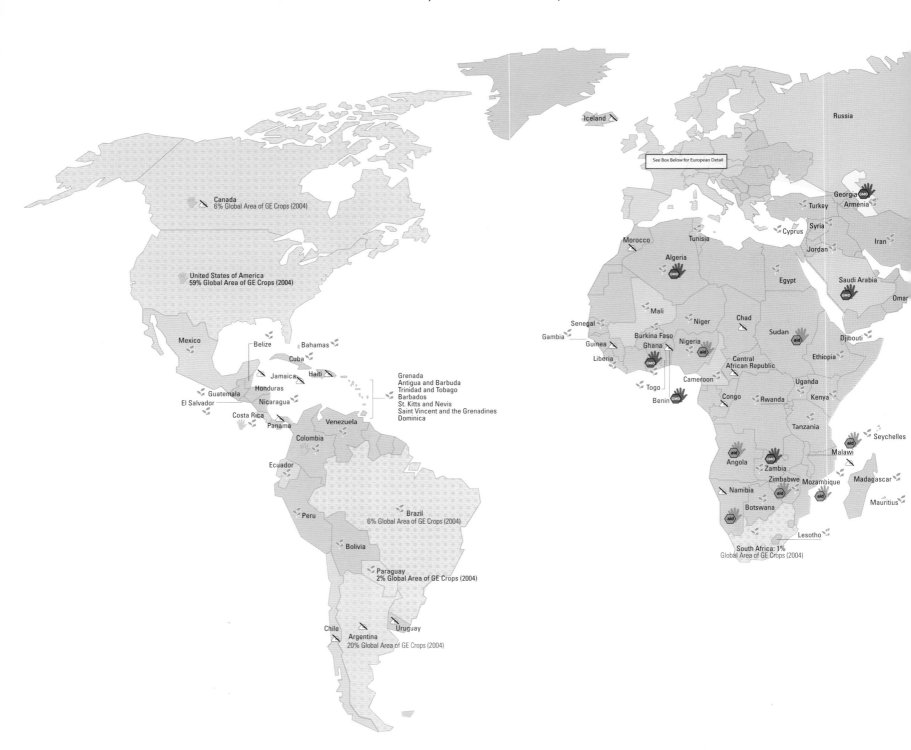

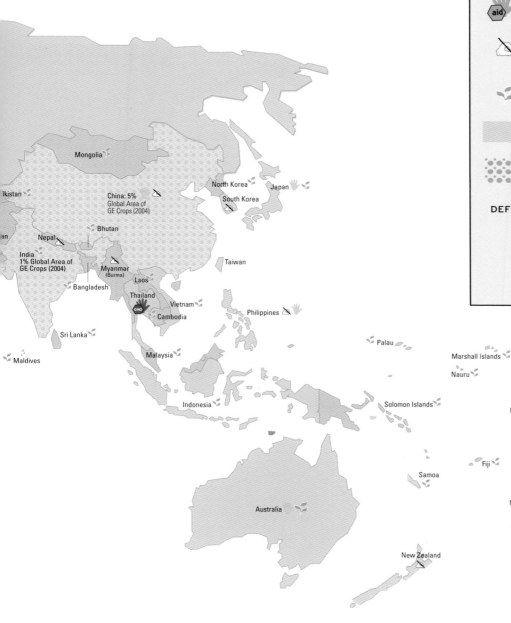

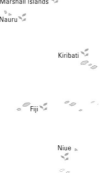

MAP LEGEND

Ban or moratorium on GMOs. Country has declared itself GE free, with either a national ban or declaration of a moratorium.

Indicates the presence of a regional ban or declaration opposing GM crop cultivation or food. For more information, please refer to "Genetically Engineered Crops and Foods: Regional Regulation and Prohibition" posted at www.centerforfoodsafety.org/geneticall5.cfm.

Country has rejected, or has policy to reject, unmilled GM grain as food aid.

Biosafety Protocol - Signed: The Biosafety Protocol, part of the Convention on Biodiversity, was initiated at the UN Earth Summit - Rio de Janiero - in 1992. The protocol aims to ensure adequate safety in the cross border movement and use of genetically modified organisms (GMOs) that may have adverse effects on the planet's biological diversity, ecosystems, and human health. The protocol was signed by more than 130 countries in January 2000, each pledging to bring the agreement before its government for ratification.

Biosafety Protocol - Ratified: The Biosafety Protocol has been ratified by governments of fifty countries (the minimum number of countries required) and thus is the first legally binding international agreement governing the movement of GMOs across national borders.

Required Labeling of GM Foods:
Country has adopted regulations requiring labeling of GM products.

Countries Cultivating GE Crops
Global Area of GE Crops (2004): USA 59%, Argentina 20%, Canada 6%, Brazil 6%, China 5%, Paraguay 2%, India 1%, South Africa 1%

DEFINITIONS

The terms "genetically modified food" or "genetically engineered food", mean food that contains or was produced with a genetically engineered or modified material.

Genetically engineered plant means a plant in which the genetic material has been changed through modern biotechnology in a way that does not occur naturally by multiplication and/or natural recombination.

Codex Alimentarius --- http://www.codexalimentarius.net

Mongolia

North Korea

Japan

South Korea

China: 5%
Global Area of
GE Crops (2004)

ikistan

Nepal

Bhutan

India
1% Global Area of
GE Crops (2004)

Myanmar
(Burma)

Taiwan

Laos

Bangladesh

Thailand

Vietnam

Cambodia

Philippines

Sri Lanka

Maldives

Malaysia

Palau

Marshall Islands

Nauru

Indonesia

Solomon Islands

Kiribati

Fiji

Samoa

Niue

Australia

New Zealand

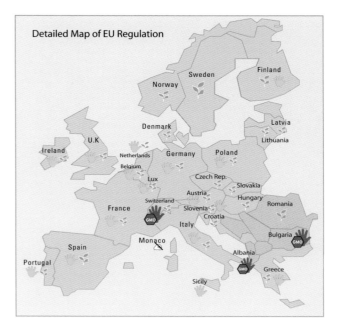

Detailed Map of EU Regulation

Norway

Sweden

Finland

Denmark

Ireland

U.K

Netherlands

Belgium

Germany

Poland

Latvia

Lithuania

Lux

Czech Rep.

Slovakia

Austria

Hungary

Romania

France

Switzerland

Slovenia

Croatia

Italy

Bulgaria

Spain

Monaco

Albania

Portugal

Sicily

Greece

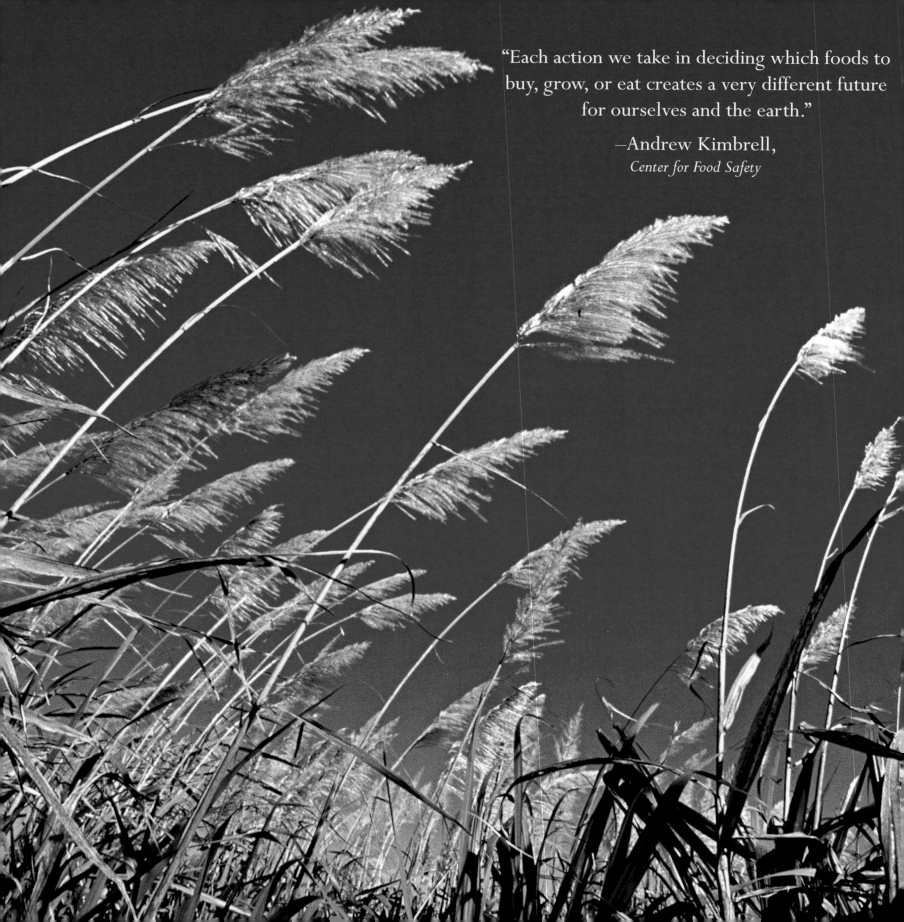

"Each action we take in deciding which foods to buy, grow, or eat creates a very different future for ourselves and the earth."

—Andrew Kimbrell,
Center for Food Safety

APPENDICES

SHOPPER'S LIST OF GE-FREE BRANDS

APPENDIX 1A

The following index is a guide for purchasing food produced without the use of genetically modified ingredients or genetically modified hormones. We list a sampling of both certified-organic lines, which are always GE-free, and brands that have made an independent pledge to exclude GE ingredients from their products. Remember that this is a partial list, and company policies can change based on the available supply of non-GE ingredients. Contact individual companies for current status, updates, and further product and distribution information.

GE-Free Grocery Store Brands

Trader Joe's brands
Whole Foods' 365 brands
Wild Oats' brands

Dairy

Certified-Organic

Horizon Organic
Organic Valley Dairy
Straus Family Creamery
Radiance Dairy
Harmony Hills Dairy
Morningland Dairy
Butterworks Farm
Stonyfield Organic Brand
Safeway Organic Brand
Alta Dena Organics
Natural by Nature
Seven Stars Farm
Wisconsin Organics

Produced Without rBGH[1]

National

Alta Dena[2]
Brown Cow Farm[3]
Lifetime Dairy[4]
Stonyfield Farms[5]
Ben & Jerry's Ice Cream[6]
Franklin County Cheese[7]
Crowley Cheese of Vermont[8]
Grafton Village Cheese[9]
Great Hill Dairy[10]

West Coast

Alpenrose Dairy[11]
Clover Stornetta Farms[12]
Joseph Farms Cheese[13]
Tillamook Cheese[14]
Berkeley Farms[15]
Wilcox Family Farms[16]
Sunshine Dairy Foods[17]

Midwest and Gulf States

Westby Cooperative Creamery[18]
Chippewa Valley Cheese[19]

Promised Land Dairy[20]
Erivan Dairy Yogurt[21]

East Coast

Crescent Creamery[22]
Blythedale Farm Cheese[23]
Erivan Dairy Yogurt[24]
Derle Farms (milk with "no rBST" label only)[25]
Farmland Dairies[26]
Wilcox Dairy (rBST-free dairy line only)[27]
Oakhurst Dairy[28]

May Be Produced Using rBGH or GE ingredients

Land O'Lakes[29]
Kemps (aside from "Select" brand)[30]
Sorrento[31]
Yoplait (General Mills)[32]
Colombo (General Mills)[33]
Parmalat[34]
Dannon[35]

Alternative Dairy Products

GE-Free:

Silk[36]

EdenSoy[37]

Imagine Foods/Soy Dream[38]

Tofutti[39]

VitaSoy/Nasoya[40]

WestSoy[41]

Belsoy[42]

Sun Soy[43]

Zen Don[44]

Pacific Soy[45]

Yves The Good Slice[46]

Nancy's Cultured Soy[47]

WholeSoy[48]

Stonyfield Farm O'Soy[49]

Soy Delicious[50]

May Contain GE Ingredients

8th Continent[51]

Eggs

GE-Free

Organic Valley

Nest Fresh Organic

Pete and Jerry's Organic Eggs

Egg Innovations Organic

Wilcox Farms Organic

Eggland's Best Organic

Land O'Lakes Organic

Baby Food & Infant Formula

GE-Free

Gerber products[52]

Earth's Best[53]

Baby's Only (certified organic products)[54]

Horizon Organic

May Contain GE Ingredients

Beech-Nut[55]

Nestlé

Good Start[56]

Similac/Isomil[57]

Enfamil[58]

Grains & Beans

GE-Free

Eden certified organic grains

Bob's Red Mill (organic line)

Vita-Spelt pasta

Annie's Natural Pasta[59]

Condiments, Oils, Dressings, & Spreads

GE-Free

Bragg's liquid amino[60]

Spectrum oils and dressings[61]

Drew's salad dressing[62]

Annie's[63]

Nasoya[64]

Muir Glen organic tomato ketchup

Maranatha Nut Butters[65]

I.M. Health™ SoyNut Butters[66]

May Contain GE Ingredients

Mazola[67]

Crisco (Smucker's)[68]

Pam (ConAgra)[69]

Wesson (ConAgra)[70]

Heinz[71]

Wish-Bone (Unilever)[72]

Kraft condiments and dressings[73]

Del Monte[74]

Hellmann's (Unilever)[75]

Smucker's (except their "Simply 100% Fruit" line of preserves)[76]

Skippy (Unilever)[77]

Peter Pan (ConAgra)[78]

Soups

GE-Free

Walnut Acres certified organic

ShariAnn's Organics

Imagine Natural[79]

Amy's Soups[80]

Fantastic Foods[81]

Health Valley/Westbrae Natural/Hain[82]

May Contain GE Ingredients

Campbell's products (including Healthy Request, Chunky, Simply Home and Pepperidge Farm)[83]

Hormel products[84]

Progresso products (General Mills)[85]

Chef Boyardee, Healthy Choice (ConAgra)[86]

Sauces/Salsas

GE-Free

Seeds of Change certified-organic pasta sauce

Walnut Acres certified-organic pasta sauce

Muir Glen Organic pasta sauce and salsa

Green Mountain certified-organic salsa

Annie's Natural[87]

May Contain GE Ingredients

Ragú (Unilever)[88]

Prego (Campbell's)[89]

Classico (Heinz)[90]

Bertolli (Unilever)[91]

Healthy Choice (ConAgra)[92]

Hunt's (ConAgra)[93]
Del Monte[94]
Chi-Chi's (Hormel)[95]
Old El Paso (General Mills)[96]
Pace (Campbell's)[97]

Canned Foods

GE-Free

Westbrae certified organic beans
ShariAnn's certified organic beans
Amy's Kitchen[98]
Annie's Natural[99]
Yves Veggie Cuisine (Hain Celestial)[100]

May Contain GE Ingredients

Chef Boyardee (ConAgra)[101]
Dinty Moore, Stagg, Hormel (Hormel)[102]
Franco-American (Campbell's)[103]

Frozen Foods

GE-Free

Linda McCartney frozen meals[104]
Barbara's Certified Organic[105]
Cascadian Farms Organic frozen meals and vegetables[106]
Amy's Kitchen[107]
A.C. LaRocco[108]
Cedarlane[109]

May Contain GE Ingredients

Tombstone (Kraft)[110]
Celeste (Pinnacle Foods)[111]
Totino's (Smucker's)[112]
Swanson (Campbell's)[113]
Stouffer's (Nestlé)[114]
Rosetto Frozen Pasta (Nestlé)[115]
Voila! (Birds Eye / Unilever)[116]

Green Giant frozen meals (General Mills)[117]
Eggo Waffles (Kellogg)[118]
Kid's Cuisine (ConAgra)[119]
Marie Callender's (ConAgra)[120]
Lean Cuisine (Nestlé)[121]
Healthy Choice (ConAgra)[122]
Morningstar Farms, Morningstar Farms Natural Touch—unless labeled organic (Kellogg)[123]
Boca—unless labeled organic (Kraft)[124]
Gardenburger[125]
Weight Watchers (Heinz)[126]
Banquet (ConAgra)[127]

Packaged Meals

GE-Free

Annie's Homegrown certified organic macaroni & cheese [128]
Seeds of Change certified organic boxed meals
Lundberg Farms Rice Sensations[129]
Casbah (Hain-Celestial)[130]
Fantastic Foods[131]
Amy's Kitchen[132]

May Contain GE Ingredients

Kraft Macaroni & Cheese meals[133]
Betty Crocker meals (General Mills)[134]
Lipton meal packets (Unilever)[135]
Pasta Roni and Rice-A-Roni meals (Quaker)[136]
Knorr (Unilever)[137]
Near East (Quaker)[138]

Bread

GE-Free

Alvarado Street[139]
French Meadow Bakery (certified organic)
Garden of Eatin'[140]

May Contain GE Ingredients

Wonder Bread (Interstate Brands)[141]
Pepperidge Farm (Campbell's)[142]
Thomas' Bread (George Weston Bakeries)[143]

Baked Goods & Baking Supplies

GE-Free

Eden Organics
Arrowhead Mills (organic line)
Bob's Red Mill (organic line)[144]
Rumford Baking Powder[145]

May Contain GE Ingredients

Aunt Jemima (Pinnacle Foods)[146]
Betty Crocker (General Mills)[147]
Pillsbury (Smucker's)[148]
Duncan Hines (Pinnacle Foods)[149]
Calumet Baking Powder (Kraft)[150]
Hungry Jack (Smucker's)[151]

Cereal

GE-Free

Barbara's (organic line)[152]
Health Valley (organic line)[153]
EnviroKidz[154]
Nature's Path[155]
Peace Cereal Organic[156]
Cascadian Farms[157]

May Contain GE Ingredients

General Mills[158]
Kellogg[159]
Quaker[160]
Post (Kraft)[161]

Snack Foods

GE-Free

Garden of Eatin'[162]

Hain PureSnax/Hain Pure Foods[163]

Kettle Foods[164]

Newman's Own Organics and Newman's Own (except salad dressing)[165]

Bearitos/Little Bear Organics (Hain Celestial)[166]

Barbara's (organic line)

Nature's Path Organic

Health Valley[167]

May Contain GE Ingredients

Kraft (Nabisco, Nilla Wafers, Oreos, Ritz, Nutter Butter, Honey Maid, SnackWells, Teddy Grams, Wheat Thins, Triscuit)[168]

Pepperidge Farm (Campbell's)[169]

Keebler (Kellogg's)[170]

Hostess Products (Interstate Brands)[171]

FritoLay (Lay's, Ruffles, Doritos, Cheetos, Tostitos)[172]

Quaker Oats Company[173]

Pringles[174]

Energy Bars

GE-Free

Clif Bar[175]

Luna Bar[176]

Odwalla[177]

Genisoy Bars[178]

May Contain GE Ingredients

PowerBar (Nestlé)[179]

Nature Valley snack bars and granola bars (General Mills)[180]

Quaker Granola Bars[181]

Nabisco Bars (Kraft)[182]

Balance Bar[183]

Chocolate

GE-Free

Endangered Species Chocolate[184]

Newman's Own[185]

Ghirardelli Chocolate[186]

Green & Black's Organic Chocolate

May Contain GE Ingredients

Nestlé (Crunch, Kit Kat, Smarties)[187]

Hershey's[188]

Toblerone (Kraft)[189]

Candy

GE-Free

Reed's Crystallized Ginger candy (certified organic)

St. Claire Organic

Jelly Belly[190]

May Contain GE Ingredients

Nestlé[191]

Lifesaver (Kraft)[192]

Hershey's[193]

Sodas and Juices

GE-Free

After the Fall organic juices (Smucker's)[194]

Crofters Organic

Eden[195]

Santa Cruz Organic (Smucker's)

Knudsen organic juices and spritzers (Smucker's)

Walnut Acres Organic Juices

Cascadian Farm[196]

Blue Sky Organic soda

Odwalla[197]

May Contain GE Ingredients

Coca-Cola (Fruitopia, Minute Maid, Hi-C, Nestea)[198]

Pepsi (Tropicana, Frappuccino, Gatorade, SoBe, Dole)[199]

Kraft (Country Time, Kool-Aid, Crystal Light, Capri Sun, Tang)[200]

Libby's (Nestlé)[201]

Blue Sky Natural Beverage Company and Hansen Beverage Company[202]

Hawaiian Punch, Sunny Delight (Procter and Gamble)[203]

Ocean Spray[204]

TOP U.S. FOOD COMPANIES AND THEIR POLICIES ON GE INGREDIENTS

APPENDIX 1B

Many of these companies own organic brands. The following policies apply to their non-organic products only.

Kraft Foods Inc.
(Altria Foods, formerly Phillip Morris)
Three Lakes Dr.
Northfield, IL 60093
Phone: 847-646-2000 *Fax:* 847-646-6005
CEO: Roger K. Deromedi *Customer comment line:* 800-622-4726
Some Kraft brands: Kraft, Nabisco, Boca Burgers, Altoids, Jell-O, Post, Taco Bell dinner kits, Tombstone, DiGiorno, Seven Seas dressing, Maxwell House, Yuban, Sanka, Kool-Aid, Capri Sun, Oscar Mayer, Cracker Barrel, Philadelphia cream cheese, Cheez Whiz, Baker's Chocolate, Calumet baking powder.
For a full list of brands, see *www.kraft.com/brands/namerica/us.html*
Policy: Uses GE ingredients, embraces biotechnology.
Transparency: Statement available at company website.[205]

Nestlé USA
800 N. Brand Blvd.
Glendale, CA 91203
Phone: 818-549-6000 *Fax:* 818-549-6952
CEO: Joe Weller *Customer comment line:* 800-225-2270
Some Nestlé brands: Nesquick, Nestea, Nescafé, Purina pet foods, PowerBar, Dreyer's ice cream, Stouffer's, Libby's, Juicy Juice, Carnation, Good Start infant formulas, Lean Cuisine.
For a full list, see *www.nestleusa.com/PubOurBrands/Brands.aspx*
Policy: Uses GE ingredients, defers to USDA and FDA.
Transparency: Statement available at company website.[206]

General Mills Inc.
One General Mills Blvd.
Minneapolis, MN 55426
Phone: 763-764-7600 *Fax:* 763-764-7384
CEO: Stephen W. Sanger *Customer comment line:* 800-248-7310
Some General Mills brands: Häagen-Dazs, 8th Continent, Betty Crocker, Big G Cereals, Bisquick, Bugles, Cascadian Farm, Cheerios, Chex, Forno de Minas, Frescarini, Fruit Snacks, Gardettos' Gold Medal, Green Giant, Hamburger Helper, Jus-Rol, Knack & Back, La Saltena, Latina, Lloyd's, Lucky Charms, Muir Glen, Nature Valley, Old El Paso, Pillsbury, Pop Secret, Progresso, Totino's/Jeno's, Trix, Wheaties, Yoplait/Colombo.

For a full list of brands, see
www.generalmills.com/corporate/brands/index.aspx
Policy: Uses GE ingredients, defers to USDA and FDA.
Transparency: Statement available from Consumer Services.[207]

Kellogg Co.
One Kellogg Sq.
Battle Creek, MI 49016
Phone: 269-961-2000 *Fax:* 269-961-2871
CEO: James M. Jenness *Customer comment line:* 800-962-1413
Some Kellogg's brands: Frosted Flakes, All-Bran, Apple Jacks, Banana Corn Flakes, Crispix, Froot Loops, Frosted Mini-Wheats, Fruit Harvest, Cheez-It, Pop-Tarts, Rice Krispies, Smart Start, Smorz, Special K, Keebler, Kashi, Morningstar Farms, Natural Touch, Nutri-Grain.
For a full list of brands, see
www.kelloggcompany.com/kelloggco/our_brands/index.html
Policy: Uses GE ingredients, defers to USDA and FDA.
Transparency: Statement available from Consumer Affairs Dept.[208]

H.J. Heinz Co.
600 Grant St.
Pittsburgh, PA 15219
Phone: 412-456-5700 *Fax:* 412-456-6015
CEO: William R. Johnson *Customer comment line:* 800-255-5750
Some Heinz brands: Bagel Bites, Boston Market, Catelli, Classico, EZ Marinader, Farley's, Greenseas, Guloso, Jack Daniel's grilling sauce, Linda McCartney meals, Mr. Yoshida's fine sauces, Ne-nerina, Olivine, Ore-Ida, Orlando, Plasmon, Polly Mi Chicha, Poppers, Rosetto, Smart Ones, tinytums, Wattie's, Weight Watchers, Wyler's.
For a full list of brands, see *www.heinz.com/jsp/world.jsp*
Policy: Uses GE, but seeks to avoid GE ingredients.
Transparency: Statement available from Consumer Resource Center.[209]

PepsiCo
700 Anderson Hill Rd.
Purchase, NY 10577-1444
Phone: 914-253-2000 *Fax:* 914-253-2070
CEO: Steven S. Reinemund

Customer comment line: 800-352-4477 (Frito-Lay line)
Some PepsiCo brands: Frito-Lay, Tropicana, Gatorade, Quaker, Pepsi, Mountain Dew, Slice, Lipton tea, Dole juices, Rold Gold pretzels.
For a full list of brands, see
www.pepsico.com/PEP_Company/BrandsCompanies/index.cfm
Policy: Uses GE ingredients, except Frito-Lay, which instructs its farmers not to plant GE crops.[210]
Transparency: Statements available from Customer Service department.[211]

Coca-Cola Company
One Coca-Cola Plaza
Atlanta, GA 30313
Phone: 404-676-2121 *Fax:* 404-676-6792
CEO: E. Neville Isdell *Customer comment line:* 800-GET-COKE
Some Coca Cola brands: Dasani, Minute Maid, Dr. Pepper, Sprite.
For a full list of brands, see *www2.coca-cola.com/brands/brandlist.html*
Policy: Uses GE ingredients, defers to USDA and FDA.
Transparency: Statement available from Industry and Consumer Affairs.[212]

ConAgra Foods Inc.
One ConAgra Dr.
Omaha, NE 68102-5001
Phone: 402-595-4000 *Fax:* 402-595-4707
CEO: Gary Rodkin *Customer comment line:* Each brand has its own toll-free number, find them at:
www.conagrafoods.com/utilities/includes/faq.jsp#Consumer
Some ConAgra brands: Blue Bonnet, Butterball, Marie Callender's, Wesson, Armour, Banquet, Chef Boyardee, Healthy Choice, Hunt's, Orville Redenbacher's, PAM, Slim Jim, Manwich, Jiffy Pop, Kid Cuisine, Egg Beaters, Reddi-wip, Knott's Berry Farm, Van Camp's.
For a full list of brands, see *www.conagrafoods.com/brandfinder/index.jsp*
Policy: Uses GE ingredients, defers to USDA and FDA.
Transparency: Statement available from Consumer Affairs.[213]

Campbell Soup Company
One Campbell Place
Camden, NJ 08103
Phone: 856-342-4800 *Fax:* 856-342-3878
CEO: Douglas R. Conant *Customer comment line:* 800-257-8443
Some Campbell's brands: Soups, Pepperidge Farm, Prego, V8, Franco-American, SpaghettiOs, Godiva chocolates, Pace.
For a full list of brands, see *www.campbellsoup.com/ourbrands.aspx*
Policy: Uses GE ingredients, defers to USDA and FDA.
Transparency: Statement available from Customer Support.[214]

Sara Lee Corp.
Three First National Plaza
Chicago, IL 60602-4260
Phone: 312-726-2600 *Fax:* 312-726-3712
CEO: Brenda C. Barnes
Customer comment line: Bakery 800-323-7117; Other 888-863-2975
Some Sara Lee brands: Breads and baked goods under the Sara Lee brand, Ball Park, Hillshire Farm, Jimmy Dean, Iron Kids, Earth Grains, Bimbo.
For a full list of Sara Lee brands, see *www.saralee.com/ourbrands*
Policy: Uses GE ingredients, defers to USDA, FDA, and EPA.
Transparency: Statement available from Public Affairs Department.[215]

The Hershey Company
100 Crystal A Dr.
Hershey, PA 17033-0810
Phone: 717-534-6799 *Fax:* 717-534-6760
CEO: Richard H. Lenny *Customer comment line:* 800-539-0261
Some Hershey's brands: Almond Joy, Breath Savers, Bubble Yum,
5th Avenue, Good & Plenty, Heath, assorted Hershey's chocolates, Ice Breakers, Jolly Rancher, Kit Kat, Milk Duds, Mounds, Payday, Reese's, Twizzlers, York, Whoppers.
For a full list of brands, see *www.hersheys.com/products*
Policy: Uses GE ingredients, defers to USDA and FDA.
Transparency: Statement available from Public Affairs Department.[216]

Hormel Foods Corp.
1 Hormel Place
Austin, MN 55912
Phone: 507-437-5611 *Fax:* 507-437-5129
CEO: Jeffrey Ettinger *Customer comment line:* 800-523-4635
Some Hormel brands: Dinty Moore, Herb-Ox, Spam, Stagg, Jennie-O turkey products, Cure 81 hams, Always Tender fresh pork, Chi-Chi's, Herdez Mexican foods, Carapelli olive oil.
For a full list of brands, see *www.hormel.com/brands/brandlist.asp*
Policy: Uses GE ingredients, defers to USDA, FDA, and EPA, and embraces biotechnology.
Transparency: Statement available from Customer Service Department.[217]

Unilever USA
800 Sylvan Avenue
Englewood Cliffs, NJ 07632
CEO: President, Unilever Americas, John Rice
Customer comment line: 877-995-4483
Some Unilever brands: Ragú, Shedd's Country Crock, I Can't Believe It's Not Butter, Wish-Bone, Skippy, Lawry's, Ben & Jerry's, Breyers, Good Humor, Bertolli, Healthy Heart, Knorr, Birds Eye, Heart, Lipton, Family Brand, Hellmann's/Bestfoods, Slim-Fast.
For a full list of brands, see *www.unileverusa.com/ourbrands/foods*
Policy: Uses GE ingredients, defers to USDA and FDA.
Transparency: Statement available at company's website.[218]

Dean Foods Co.
2515 McKinney Ave., Ste. 1200
Dallas, TX 75201
Phone: 214-303-3400 *Fax:* 214-303-3499
CEO: Gregg L. Engles *Customer comment line:* Listed on individual brand packages.
Some Dean Foods brands: Silk, AltaDena, Barber's, Berkeley Farms, Borden, Brown's Dairy, Country Delite, Country Fresh, Creamland, Hershey's Milk, Land O'Lakes, LehighValley, Meadow Brook, Meadow Gold, PET, Reiter, Robinson, Schenkel's, Schepps, Shenandoah's, Swiss, T.G. Lee, Tuscan, Verifine, Horizon Organic, Rachel's Organic, Marie's dressings, Stroh's, Oak Farms, Morning Sun, Flap Jack, Happy Kids, Carb Conquest, Folgers Jakada, Healthy Shake.
For a full list of products, see *www.deanfoods.com/brands/brands.asp*
Policy: Varies by brand.

Flowers Foods Inc.
1919 Flowers Cir.
Thomasville, GA 31757
Phone: 229-226-9110 *Fax:* 229-225-3806
CEO: George E. Deese *Customer comment line:* Check individual products for toll-free numbers.
Some Flowers Foods brands: Nature's Own, Cobblestone Mill, Sunbeam, Bunny, Dandee, Mary Jane, ButterKrust, Bluebird, Mrs. Freshley's, European BakersFor a full list of products, see
www.flowersfoods.com/FFC_Brands/index.cfm
Policy: Uses GE ingredients.
Transparency: Statement available from Technical Services Department.[219]

GUIDE TO PROCESSED FOOD ADDITIVES
APPENDIX 1C

The laundry list of ingredients in processed foods can be overwhelming, even for the savviest of consumers. Most of the confusion arises from additives with vague or technical names that cannot be pinned easily to their source. These ambiguous ingredients pose a special challenge to the shopper attempting to avoid GE foods. Below is a partial list of additives that are sometimes derived from GE crops. Watch out for these sneaky ingredients on your next trip to the grocery store.[220]

Soy-derived additives:

Soy flour

Soy isolate

Soy isoflavones

Soy lecithin

Soy protein

Soybean oil

Corn-derived additives:

Corn flour

Corn masa

Cornmeal

Corn oil

Cornstarch

Corn syrup

High fructose corn syrup

Vanilla extract (contains corn syrup)

Additives with multiple sources (may be derived from corn, soy, or another source):

Ascorbate (Vitamin C)

Aspartame

Beta-carotene (pro-Vitamin A)

Caramel

Carotenoids

Cellulose

Cobalamin (Vitamin B12)

Cystein

Dextrin

Dextrose

Fructose

Glucose

Glutamate

Gluten

Hemicellulose

Inositol

Invert sugars

Lactose

Lactoflavin

Leucine

Lysine

Maltose

Methionine

Methylcellulose

Modified starch

Mono- and diglycerides

Monosodium glutamate (MSG)

Niacin

Phenylalanine

Riboflavin (Vitamin B2)

Sorbitol

Textured Vegetable Protein (TVP)

Threonine

Tocopherol (Vitamin E)

Tryptophan

Vegetable fat

Vegetable oil

Xanthan gum

Zein

COMMUNITY ORGANIZING GUIDE
APPENDIX 2A

"If you want to move people, it has to be toward a vision that's positive for them, that taps important values, that gets them something they desire, and it has to be presented in a compelling way that they feel inspired to follow." — *Martin Luther King, Jr.*

Recruitment is possibly the most important and overlooked part of organizing. People by nature want to feel involved in something. Recruiting volunteers and members is a great way to develop your group and to help people fulfill their desires to act for positive change. People join groups for several reasons, and usually, all you have to do is ask them to join. If you have shared values and vision, a strong campaign and something that relates to their community, you are sure to get volunteers. When you talk to people about joining your group, always emphasize the issues that matter to them. Are they parents? Teachers? Healthcare workers? Find out why this issue is important to them. Recruiting, like so many other aspects of organizing, comes down to relationships. Don't spend so much time telling them why they should care about your issue; instead, spend that time finding out why it matters to them.

Planning Action in your Community

People join groups for a number of reasons:
•To address issues that affect their community.
•To act on their morals, ethics, values, and visions.
•To meet like-minded people.
•To have fun.
Some tips on how to recruit: Outreach should be built into every aspect of your campaign. Your group should be doing consistent activities that raise the recognition of the group while giving people the opportunity to join. This is easily accomplished at tabling and petitioning events.

Your group can also plan a teach-in on the issue or hold a larger public event just to draw a bigger crowd and see who is interested in joining. You can also do this at related events planned by other groups— many will let you have a table with information at their event. At each event, ask every interested person if he or she wants to volunteer. You should have simple tasks for your volunteers. Usually, if one person out of ten shows up to volunteer, you are doing well.

Recruit for an activity or an event—not another meeting. You want people involved who are active and want to be active; avoid chronic meeting-goers. If all that your group offers is meetings, new people will drop out. There is nothing wrong with occasional meetings to bring everyone together and talk about how the campaign is going, but don't rely on these meetings as the bulk of your activities. Recruit people to run a table on weekends, start a petition drive in their community, speak at their child's PTA meeting, or make a presentation at their local place of worship.

Delegate responsibilities. César Chávez once said the organizer's job is to help ordinary people do extraordinary things. No one person in the group should be responsible for recruiting and coordinating volunteers. One idea is to have new members or volunteers run the tables or petitioning activities where they were recruited. They are familiar with the activity and know it can be done. This in turn develops a sense of involvement and leadership.

Be inspired and inspiring. If you are motivated and inspired by the group and campaign, you will be motivating and inspiring to others.

Listen to people. The best leaders are those who spend more time listening and asking questions rather than talking at people. Good recruiting is based on conversation; avoid reciting a monologue on the wonder of your work. You need to be able to draw people out. What are their interests? Why do they care about this issue? Remember that listening is active.

Get a commitment and follow it up. Get people to commit to a certain activity on a specified day. Let them know you will follow up with them between now and the scheduled time—tell them what day you will call, who will call, etc. Be clear about the subsequent plan. Then call them when you said you would call. Following up is very important. This lets new volunteers know the group is organized, does what it says it will, and that people really do want their involvement. When they show up at the event, make a point of welcoming them and including them in decision-making.

Develop leaders from volunteers. Once you've recruited people the next step is to involve them at a higher level. To develop leaders, get to know people's strengths and weaknesses. What do they enjoy doing? What are they good at? Think through what the group needs, and come up with a plan on how to develop new people to the next level (e.g., from petitioning to petitioning coordinator, from attending the news conference to learning how to write the news release). Developing leaders takes time and training; making this investment at the outset will ultimately benefit your campaign. If the group doesn't have the time to train, call around to other groups that might be willing to offer some instruction. Check out the resources section of this book for organizations.

Recruiting and maintaining new members in your group is not only essential, it's fun and exciting too!

Organizing a Meeting

Hosting a meeting of like-minded people could be your first step in community outreach. Your action will be more effective with even a small group working together. Reach out to friends, neighbors, classmates—anyone who you think would be interested in learning more and getting active. Look for allies at natural food stores, restaurants, local nature centers, farmers' markets, alternative health centers—anywhere people are concerned about food, health, or the environment.

Publicize the meeting. Use e-mails, fliers, and announcements in event calendars. Written announcements should be followed up with phone calls to remind people of the meeting.

Plan the meeting. Have clear goals and an agenda with time scheduled for each agenda item. Invite a facilitator to focus the group on the agenda and to encourage participation. Enlist a timekeeper to keep the meeting on schedule and a meeting secretary to keep minutes.

Start and stop the meeting on time. If meetings perpetually start late, people will stop showing up on time or at all. Time is precious these days, so start and stop on time.

Have a sign-in sheet. Use the sheet to collect contact information from everyone. Make it available so people can stay in touch.

Break the ice. Plan a fun, relaxing start to the meeting. Begin the meeting with introductions. Have everyone say something about him or herself and why he or she is interested in the issue. Before starting, the group should reach a common understanding for meeting process. For example, decide whether people should raise hands or jump in to talk.

Prepare an agenda. After introductions and common understandings, you'll get to the "business" of the meeting. "Brainstorming" can be a useful tool: this means exploring ideas from everyone in the group, without allowing any discussion or judgment of whether the ideas are possible or worthwhile. Keep brainstorms to a set time, but allow flexibility if lots of ideas are coming out. Then take time to choose and prioritize ideas that the group wants to pursue. There may be subgroups; some people may want to pursue one approach while others prefer another. It's also a good idea to have some action people can take at the meeting—for example, write a letter to the store manager of your local supermarket store, a letter to your Representative or Senator, or a letter to the editor. This makes people feel part of an active community.

Get commitments. By the end of the meeting have an action plan with clear agreement from people to take on certain tasks and a clear time for reporting on progress.

Follow up. Be sure to follow up with all the people who attended your meeting. Call them and thank them for coming; send out reminders for any action people agreed to take; remind people about any upcoming events your group planned; and keep them involved. It is also a good idea to contact the people you invited who didn't attend. Let them know what happened at the meeting and encourage their attendance at the next activity. This will help them feel more involved in the group.

Start Organizing

Any one of the suggestions below would be a good start to your organizing:
• Plan a tabling or petitioning event.
• Plan a meeting with managers from a local supermarket.
• Plan a supermarket tour.
• Organize outreach to local media; set up groups to write letters to the editor and make calls to talk radio stations. (See "Community Media Guide.")
• Plan other educational events in the community: link with schools, fairs or other community organizations.

Planning a Tabling or Petitioning Event

Setting up a table with the group's information is a great way to accomplish campaign goals and engage the public. While tabling, you can get petitions signed, letters written, and volunteers signed up. Here are some tips to great tabling:

• If you plan to set up the table in front of a store, ask the manager first for permission. You may be told you cannot be on their property; however, in many cases there is a public sidewalk or shopping center thoroughfare where you can legally set up your table. If you don't know, check with your local police department or an attorney to find out what your rights are in that particular space and whether or not you need a permit. If you are asked to leave and are unsure of your rights, you should leave.
• Try to have at least two people to run the table. This makes it more fun than standing there by yourself. It is also easier to engage people if you have one person standing behind the table and one nearby with a clipboard of petitions and fliers.
• Set up your table in a spot where you will not block the flow of customer foot and automobile traffic.
• Make sure you have materials. For fliers, petitions, and other printable resources, visit www.truefoodnow.org and www.centerforfoodsafety.org
• Be sure to have a sign-up sheet for those interested in volunteering or coming to the next meeting or event.
• A good activity at a table is having people write letters to the company, city council member, or decision-maker you're targeting. Have a short sample letter on hand and paper on which to write. (See the sample letter on page 130.) Keep these letters and mail them for people. This ensures they are actually delivered.
• Petitions are an easy way to get people interested in your campaign and make their voices heard too. You should set a goal for the number of signatures you want to collect before you send them in. Work out how many hours a week your group will need to spend collecting signatures to reach that goal. The petitions can then be saved until you get the number of signatures you've set as your campaign goal, or you can send them as they come in at strategic moments in your campaign.

Tabling Checklist

1. Fliers
2. Petitions, postcards, sample letters—whatever you choose
3. Volunteer sign-up sheets
4. A sign or banner with the name of your group
5. Pens... lots of pens
6. Clipboards—these help the volunteers walking around with petitions and keep materials on the table from blowing away
7. A donation can

Again, follow-up is key. Promptly call anyone who signed up to volunteer and involve them in the next event. As you enlist more volunteers, set up a phone tree to remind everyone to come out as scheduled and include more people in the recruitment process.

Planning a Meeting with Store Management, Potential Allies, or Elected Officials

Once you have scheduled a meeting with store management, potential allies, or elected officials, you should begin planning. Go into the meeting with a specific request in mind:

• Ask supermarkets to assure you that their store brands are made without GE ingredients.
• Ask them to request policies from their suppliers, ensuring they will source only non-GE ingredients for the products they make for the supermarket.
• Ask allies to help spread the word, to display literature, to print an article on your campaign in their group newsletter, to host a meeting in their community, or to help plan and attend your group's events.
• Ask elected officials to support a specific bill, regulation, or policy. Ask them to put pressure on the FDA, USDA, and EPA.

Meeting Tips

•Each member of your group should have something to say in the meeting. Keep it brief, but give each person a chance to speak.
•Bring background material; assume the person you are meeting with knows nothing about the issue. Bring fact sheets and articles that make your main points.
•Be polite. A meeting is the start of a relationship. The person you meet with may not agree or do what you want. Your follow-up—whether it's organizing a demonstration or another meeting with more people—is just as important as the meeting itself and can lead to further communication down the road.
•If you are asked a question you can't answer, be honest. Offer to get back to the person later on.
•Phone the people you met with a week or so afterwards to see whether or not they've made any progress on their commitments.
•Keep your group informed of any developments, and be ready to act if agreements are not upheld.

Planning a Supermarket Tour

Supermarket tours can be done wherever you live to raise the consciousness of markets and consumers alike. Tours are not a demonstration or protest, but a way to engage shoppers and store personnel in learning about genetically engineered (GE) ingredients in our food and GE crops in our environment. The goal of the tour is to increase awareness of GE foods and begin a process of engagement with the store. You and your group can help empower others to raise consumer concerns about GE foods in your area stores.

Advance Planning

Choose a major chain, preferably one that sells its own store-brand products (for example, Safeway Select and Lucerne are two store brands of Safeway, Dominick's, and other affiliated stores). If it's not your neighborhood store, visit the target market often enough to give you a good feel for its layout, inside and out.

Advertise the supermarket tour, widely and well in advance. Remember to invite local church and civic leaders, politicians, chefs, restaurant owners, teachers and students, as well as vegetarian, senior citizen, and environmental groups. It's also very important to invite gardeners and farmers, especially organic food producers and food co-op organizers.

Contact the supermarket manager a few days before you plan to conduct the tour. Explain what you intend to do and why. Invite store personnel to take part in the tour. You should be prepared for the store management not to allow your tour. In that case, you can proceed with your plans, but be ready if store management confronts you. Be clear that you and your group are shoppers and want to discuss issues while you shop; reassure the store management that you will not block aisles, speak loudly, or otherwise impair other shoppers. If they still refuse, set up your information table outside and ask your group to pass out fliers and gather signatures on petitions. You should also ask how to contact the store's regional or national management to complain about being barred from that store.

Contact your city government beforehand to find out where you can table on public ground near the store (usually sidewalks along storefronts are public ground, but check to see if you need a permit). Plan your route through the store and prepare your script.

The Tour Day

Outside the supermarket

Set up your information table outside and as close to the market entrance as possible. You may have to investigate your legal rights to public space, as noted above.

Have your table stocked with printed handouts and a clipboard for collecting signatures and the names and addresses of participants and interested passersby. Have a friendly, courteous volunteer or two ready to talk about GE foods.

At tour time, assemble your participants. Introduce yourself. Thank them for coming and brief them on what to expect inside the store. Encourage tour members to ask questions, of you and of store personnel. Make sure everyone has copies of fact sheets and other material. The tour leader should carry additional leaflets to give people who join the tour or seem interested.

Inside the Supermarket

Ideally you should have two people, a tour guide and a traffic manager, conduct the tour. The guide leads the tour and speaks at each station. The traffic manager follows the group, keeps it together and invites other shoppers to join the tour.

Speak confidently and clearly. Be friendly and determined. This is easiest if you're well prepared with a script in hand.

Become familiar with the company policies included in Appendix 1B. Be ready to point out which brands use or avoid GMOs, without overly praising or blaming specific companies. If you don't know a company's policy or if other tough questions come up, urge tour members to ask the store manager and call the company's toll-free number.

Sample Letter to Supermarket Management

[Store Name]
[Date]
[Name of manager]
[Store management]

Dear_____,

I am a loyal shopper and I am writing today to ask that your supermarket eliminate the use of genetically engineered (GE) ingredients in your store-brand products. Your customers shop in your stores because we expect high-quality foods that are good for our families. The continued use of GE ingredients in your store brands undermines my confidence in the quality of your products.

I am concerned about GE foods because... [in this paragraph, describe in your own words why you are concerned. For instance: corporate control of the food supply, genetic contamination of organic crops, human health risks, lack of choice, etc.] In response to the threat of GE foods, I urge you to do the right thing: remove genetically engineered ingredients from your store-brand products. By making this commitment, your store is protecting the health of your customers and of the environment. Three national chains, Trader Joe's, Whole Foods, and Wild Oats, have already made this commitment.

I am deeply disappointed that [supermarket name] has so far failed to take action to protect its customers from these unlabeled GE foods. Since I do not want to buy genetically engineered foods, I hope that you will eliminate GE ingredients in your store-brand products so I can feel confident about shopping in your store.

Sincerely,
[your name and address]

COMMUNITY ORGANIZING RESOURCES
APPENDIX 2B

Community Get-togethers

Eat Grub – Organic community dinner parties are loads of fun!
www.eatgrub.org

Earth Dinner – It's not just for Earth Day! Ideas, cards, recipes, and more. *www.earthdinner.org.*

Host a movie party – Organic Consumers Association has a good list of films and ideas. *www.organicconsumers.org/films.htm.*

Start a GE-Free or Organic Meetup group – Organize a "Meetup" at your favorite farmers market or organic restaurant! *www.meetup.com*

Organizing Skills and Training

GEAN (Genetic Engineering Action network)
National network of grassroots groups, offers grassroots skills and trainings on GE issues and an annual national conference including trainings and workshops. *www.geaction.org* 617-661-6626

MidWest Academy
Offers training sessions for leaders and staff of community groups. *www.midwestacademy.com.*

Green Corps
National field school for environmental grassroots organizing. Offers a one-year program for recent college graduates. *www.greencorps.org*

Books:
Rules for Radicals: A Pragmatic Primer for Realistic Radicals, Alinsky, Saul D., New York: Vintage Books, 1971.

Organizing for Social Change, MidWest Academy, Santa Ana, CA: Seven Locks Press, 2001. 800-354-5348 or *www.mindspring/~midwestacademy/Book/page3.html*

The Activist's Handbook: A Primer for the 1990s and Beyond, Shaw, Randy, Berkeley: University of California Press, 1996.

Fundraising

Books:
Environmental Grantmaking Foundations, Corrine R. Szymko, ed., Resources for Global Sustainability, 800-724-1857.

Fundraising for Social Change, Kim Klein, Chardon Press, P.O. Box 101, Inverness, CA 94937, $20.00.

Grantseeker's Guide,
James McGrath Morris and Laura Adler, eds., Moyer Bell, Colonial Hill/RFD 1, Mt. Kisco, NY 10549, $39.95

Grassroots Grants: An Activist's Guide to Proposal Writing, Andy Robinson, Chardon Press, P.O. Box 101, Inverness, CA 94937, $25.00

The Grassroots Fundraising Book,
Joan Flanagan, The Youth Project, 2335 18th St. NW, Washington, D.C. 20009, $8.95.

The Whole Nonprofit Catalog,
The Grantsmanship Center. P.O. Box 17220, Los Angeles, CA 90017. This catalog is free.

Websites
The Foundation Center:
www.foundationcenter.org

National Committee for Responsive Philanthropy:
www.ncrp.org

The Environmental Support Center:
www.envsc.org

Community Media Guide

Using the media is a great way to raise awareness about genetic engineering, apply pressure to the target of your campaign, and build name recognition and strength for your group. It is a good idea to strategically incorporate media events into your campaign timeline. When to call the press is largely dependent on your campaign goals; however, there are some frequently used media tactics.

Contact the media:
• When you announce your campaign or program.
• At key times such as local elections or regulatory comment periods.
• When you can link your campaign to current local news.
• To release a report or new information about the campaign or the campaign target.
• When you have a big event such as a large public rally or community meeting.

Keep in mind that calling the media to talk solely about your campaign rarely works.

You also need to have an event to bring them out. Remember, reporters are concerned about getting a good story that is relevant to their readers or viewers and that sells papers and airtime. Even print reporters are relying more and more on the visual aspects of an event, so be sure you have something good for them to see. Even if they don't run a photo they will often describe the scene in their story. Look at the pictures and read the descriptions of the "scene" in recent local stories to get a better sense of this. Think about what you want the "picture" to look like in advance. What message are you conveying? Is the name of your group in a prominent place? Even if you don't plan on it, you may attract the press by your action against genetic engineering, so be prepared.

Developing Relationships with the Press

It pays to do some research into local media before your event. Keep track of who writes the consumer stories, the environmental stories, and the progressive business stories. Study the writing style of each reporter or newspaper. When you have an event, call the assignment or news desk and find out who covers that particular beat. After a while, you will know which reporter to contact. As you develop a good media list, set up a database of your contacts to make faxing and e-mailing easier. Make sure to include personal notes in the database that will help you identify each person later. Keep the contact consistent. It's a good idea to designate one person to handle all the media contact, including press releases and advisories.

Working with the media often comes down to relationships. Follow up with the journalist after he or she covers your event. Don't harass

the reporter, but build up a rapport to keep him or her interested in your campaign. It is also helpful to occasionally send cooperative reporters news clips or press releases on issues related to your campaign. Don't overwhelm them, but give them the background they need to write an informed story. As reporters come to trust you as a source, they will call you when the issue comes up again and use your knowledge for attribution. Always send a thank you note to a reporter who has done a good job covering the story. And don't be afraid to call a reporter who has the facts wrong or misquoted you—papers will run corrections.

The Press Advisory

If you want to invite the press to cover your local event, you will need to let reporters know ahead of time by writing a press advisory. This alerts reporters to the basics: the who, what, why, where, when, and how of your event. You should fax or e-mail it, and then call to make sure the reporter received the advisory and to find out whether or not he is planning to attend.

Press Advisory Tips:
• The advisory is intended to serve as a notice to the media about your upcoming event. It is meant to entice the media without giving away the whole story.
• The headline and first lines of the advisory are critical. Busy reporters will only read the headline and maybe the first sentence of the advisory to decide whether or not they'll cover the event.
• News advisories should be short—no more than a half page.
• Advisories should be sent out one to two days before the event.
• Never assume the media has seen your advisories after you've faxed or e-mailed them. Call to follow up.
• Press calls should be made the day the advisories are sent out and again the day of the event.
• If a print reporter commits to attending the event, don't contact him or her again unless you have new information. This is a judgment call, but you do not want to ruin relationships with the media by hounding your contacts.

Excellent Visuals

Sample Press Advisory

CALL FOR END OF GENETICALLY MODIFIED FOODS IN SUPERMARKET'S PRODUCTS WOMEN. PARENT GROUPS TAKE ACTION AT FOOD RETAILER

WHAT: The coalition is calling on Safeway to end its use of genetically engineered ingredients in its store brand products. A coalition of women's groups and parent organizations, joined by San Jose Resistance Against GMOs, will demonstrate in front of the nationwide food retailer Wednesday.
WHEN: Wednesday, May 15th, 11 a.m.
WHERE: Safeway, 555 Main Street (at Jones Street), San Jose
WHO: Women for Safe Food, Mothers for Labeling, San Jose Parent Club, and San Jose Resistance Against GMOs
Contacts: Sally Smith of San Jose Resistance Against GMOs, 408-555-1212; John Jones of San Jose Parent Club, 408-555-1311

The Press Release

On the day of the event, send the same reporters a press release. This should include the information in your advisory (time, place, etc.), but go into more detail. Explain how the event will proceed and why you are doing it. Include the relevance of the issue and the background of your event.

Press Release Tips:

• The press release should read like a newspaper article with quotes from your spokespeople.
• Just as with the advisory, the headline and first lines of the release are critical. Busy reporters will only read the headline and maybe the first sentence.
• Ensure that the details and contacts for the event are clearly marked at the top of the release, not buried in the text or at the end.
• Keep to no more than one main message with two subordinate messages in the news release. What is the main message of the news release?
• A news release should never be longer than a page.
• Whenever possible, include links to background information, statistics, and details about the issue or event.
• Keep copies of the release along with other relevant materials (e.g., fact sheets) with you at the event as part of your press kit, and make sure you give it to reporters.
• For the media that do not attend, fax or e-mail the news release after the event and call to pitch the story.
• Below is a sample release from a fictitious event. Feel free to use this as a guide for your own release.

Sample Press Release

CALL FOR END OF GENETICALLY MODIFIED FOOD IN SAFEWAY'S PRODUCTS. WOMEN, PARENT GROUPS TAKE ACTION AT FOOD RETAILER

Contacts: Sally Smith, San Jose Parent Club, 408-555-1212, John Jones, San Jose Community Group, 408-555-1311

San Jose, May 15th—A coalition of women's groups and parent organizations, joined by San Jose Resistance Against GMOs, is calling on the food retailer to end its use of genetically engineered ingredients in its store brand products. To demonstrate their disfavor, the protesters symbolically dumped Safeway's store brand products in a garbage can marked with Biohazard tape.

"We don't want to eat genetic experiments," said Sally Smith of the San Jose Parent Club. "We want Safeway to protect our health and environment by removing genetically engineered ingredients from their store brand products."

The coalition also presented the local manager with 1,000 petition signatures collected from San Jose Safeway customers. A letter from the coalition accompanied the petitions.

The San Jose coalition is part of a national coalition of grassroots community groups calling on the retailer to change its practices.

"Safeway tells its customers they provide safe, healthy food," said John Jones of San Jose Community Group. "But there is nothing safe or healthy about genetically engineered food. It's untested, unregulated, risky food. They are doing business the Un-Safeway."

Genetic engineering creates for the first time "living pollution," bringing known and unknown risks to the environment and public health.

Unlike traditional crop breeding, genetic engineering enables scientists to cross genes from bacteria, viruses, and animals into plants. The risks include the creation of new food allergies, superweeds, and increased toxic herbicide use. Additionally, the gene-altered corn found in the Safeway product contains an antibiotic resistant marker gene that science and medical organizations, including the British Medical Association, warn could make some common antibiotics useless.

"Safeway customers have clearly spoken," said Smith. "When we were petitioning Safeway customers they were surprised to hear that the company uses genetically engineered ingredients. People just don't want to eat GE foods."

At the same time of today's action, the Los Angeles group GE-Free LA held a food dump in front of a Los Angeles Von's store, a subsidiary of Safeway.

Interviews

If you get reporters to come to your event, they will want to hear your story. You should have a media spokesperson or two from your group chosen before the event. Everyone attending your event should know who these spokespeople are and be able to point them out to the reporters. Prepare one or two lines—also known as soundbites—which you go over in advance so everyone knows the message that you want to get across to the press. This is important because the press will likely want to talk to as many people as possible. Most reporters want to hear directly from the people most affected by the issue. Be sure to have these people available and prepared to answer questions.

Spokespeople should be prepared ahead of time with short, clear answers to common questions. For television or radio in particular, soundbites are likely to be all the reporter can use, so keep each point to ten to fifteen seconds. Be careful what you say; be prepared with your arguments and stick to them. For example, if a reporter says, "Isn't it true that there's no evidence that GE food has harmed anyone?" you might respond, "GE food hasn't harmed anyone but we don't know what the long-term threat is." The next day you might be misquoted like this: "Jim Green of CAGE agreed that 'GE foods haven't harmed anyone.'" A better answer is: "There is no evidence that GE foods are safe in the long run, yet they are not labeled so we can't avoid eating them." You can also ask the reporter to e-mail you questions. That way you can word your responses with care and you'll have a written copy of your correspondence.

Use positive language as much as possible. Don't just say, "We oppose GE food." Reframe your answer as "We support the consumer's right to know what's in our food and to choose food made without GE ingredients." If a question comes up that you can't answer, it's okay to tell the reporter you don't know. You can always look into the matter and get back to him. This is always preferable to making something up which could come back to haunt you.

Media Follow-Up

Be sure to collect contact information from any reporters who attend your event or who interview you by phone. Exchange business cards whenever possible. Assign a media coordinator at your event to ensure that all reporters and photographers are greeted, given a press kit, and signed in on a media contact sheet. You can also supply nametags to your attendees so that reporters can easily identify them by name and title.

The success of media coverage usually comes down to how well your campaign conveys a problem faced by many people in the community.

The goal is to engage participants in the debate of that problem. Remember that "any press is good press" so don't get discouraged by a few bad quotes or low-media attendance. If people are talking about the issue, if it's being debated in the press, in schools, in supermarkets, and in homes, your media work is a success.

Event Preparations:
• Will you need a microphone, podium, or other public address system?
• Have you recruited a good number of volunteers to be at the event?
• Who is sending out the press advisory?
• Who is making follow-up phone calls?
• Do you have good visuals arranged for your event? How will you create dynamic shots to engage photographers and reporters?
• Do you have good soundbites (short quotes) memorized?
• Does everyone know who the media spokesperson is?
• Do you need a translator?
• Do you have answers ready for questions you expect to get from the press? (e.g., Why are you here today? What do you want _____ to do? Isn't GE food okay by the FDA?)
• Who is sending the press release?
• Who is making follow-up calls?

Press Kit Checklist
1. Background information on the issue and your campaign, including fact sheets.
2. Information on any speakers and their backgrounds, organizations, etc.
3. Copies of statements made at the event, any reports released.
4. A copy of the press release.
5. People and websites to contact with further questions.

Writing Letters to the Editor
One thing you can do make your voice heard is to write a letter to the editor. Typically, you should begin your letter by referencing the article (with publication date) to which you are responding. Call the paper to check the guidelines and maximum number of words—some require fewer than 150, some will accept up to 500 words.

Tips:
•Keep it to one concise point/criticism of the article you are writing in response to.
•Try to shed light on an angle that the article didn't cover.
•Explain how the issue the article talks about may impact your local area. Readers will always be more interested in something that they think may directly affect their community.
•Don't assume readers are informed on your issue. Give a concise yet informative background before launching into your main point.
•When possible, include data to back your argument.
•Always provide contact information. Most papers won't print anonymous letters.

Media Resources:

Spin Project (The Strategic Press Information Network)
Provides media technical assistance to nonprofit public-interest organizations. *www.spinproject.org*

Media Alliance
A nonprofit training center for media workers, community organizations, and political activists. *www.media-alliance.org*

FAIR (Fairness and Accuracy in Reporting)

Offers a media guide for activists. *www.fair.org/activism/activismkit.html*

Green Media Toolshed
Provides media tools, media training, online pressroom, image management, and a media database. *www.greenmediatoolshed.org*

ORGANIZATIONS AND WEB RESOURCES
APPENDIX 3A

Genetic Engineering —
National

Alliance for Bio-Integrity
2040 Pearl Ln., Ste. 2
Fairfield, IA 52556
Phone: 641-469-2048
www.biointegrity.org

Amberwaves
305 Brooker Hill Rd. Box 487
Becket, MA 01223
Phone: 413-623-0012
www.amberwaves.org

The Campaign to Label GE Foods
(The Campaign)
P.O. Box 55699
Seattle, WA 98155
Phone: 425-771-4049
www.thecampaign.org

Center for Food Safety
660 Pennsylvania Ave. S.E., Ste. 302
Washington, D.C. 20003
Phone: 202-547-9359
www.centerforfoodsafety.org

Center for Ethics and Toxics
P.O. Box 673
39120 Ocean Dr., Ste. C-2-1
Gualala, CA 95445
Phone: 707- 884-1700
www.cetos.org

Consumers Union
101 Truman Ave.
Yonkers, NY 10703-1057
Phone: 914-378-2000
www.consumersunion.org

Council for Responsible Genetics
5 Upland Rd., Ste. 3
Cambridge, MA 02140
Phone: 617-868-0870
www.gene-watch.org

Edmonds Institute
20319-92nd Ave. West
Edmonds, WA 98020
Phone: 425-775-5383
www.edmonds-institute.org

Environmental Defense
257 Park Ave. South
New York, NY 10010
Phone: 212-505-2100
www.environmentaldefense.org

Foundation on Economic Trends
4520 East West Hwy., Ste. 600
Bethesda, MD 20814
Phone: 301-656-6272
www.foet.org

Free the Planet!
218 D St. S.E.
Washington D.C. 20003
Phone: 202-547-3656
www.freetheplanet.org

Friends of the Earth
1717 Massachusetts Ave. N.W., Ste. 600
Washington, D.C. 20036-2002
Phone: 877-843-8687 (toll-free)
www.foe.org/safefood

Genetic Engineering
Action Network
P.O. Box 194
Mechanicsville, IA 52306
Phone: 563-432-6735
www.geaction.org

Institute for Agriculture
and Trade Policy
2105 First Ave. South
Minneapolis, MN 55404
Phone: 612-870-0453
www.iatp.org

Institute for Social Ecology
1118 Maple Hill Rd.
Plainfield, VT 05667
Phone: 802-454-8493
www.biodev.org

Mothers for Natural Law
P.O. Box 1177
Fairfield, IA 52556
www.safe-food.org

National Family Farm Coalition
110 Maryland Ave. N.E., Ste. 307
Washington, D.C. 20002
Phone: 202-543-5675
www.nffc.net
(See the Farmers Declaration on Genetic
Engineering in Agriculture.)

Oakland Institute
P.O. Box 18978
Oakland, CA 94619
www.oaklandinstitute.org

PCC Natural Markets
4201 Roosevelt Way N.E.
Seattle, WA 98105
Phone: 206-547-1222
www.pccnaturalmarkets.com/issues/ge.html

**Pew Initiative on Food
and Biotechnology**
1331 H St., Ste. 900
Washington, D.C. 20005
Phone: 202-347-9044
httz://pweagbiotech.org

Sierra Club
85 Second St., Second Floor
San Francisco, CA 94105
Phone: 415-977-5500
www.sierraclub.org/biotech

The True Food Network
Grassroots Network for
the Center of Food Safety
2601 Mission Street, Suite 803
San Francisco, CA 94110
Phone: 415-826-2770
www.truefoodnow.org

Union of Concerned Scientists
2 Brattle Sq.
Cambridge, MA 02238
Phone: 617-547-5552
*www.ucusa.org/food_and_environment/genetic_
engineering*

*Genetic Engineering —
Regional*

**Californians for
GE-Free Agriculture**
www.calgefree.org

GE-Free Mendocino
(Mendocino County, CA)
www.gmofreemendo.com

GE-Free Alameda (Alameda County, CA)
www.gmofreeac.org

GE-Free Sonoma (Sonoma County, CA)
www.gefreesonoma.org

GE-Free Vermont
www.gefreevt.org

Rural Vermont
www.ruralvermont.org

GE-Free Maine
www.gefreemaine.org

GMO-Free Hawai'i
www.gmofreehawaii.org

GeneWise (Chicago area)
www.genewise.org

**Oregon Physicians for Social
Responsibility**
www.oregonprs.org

SOS Food NY (New York)
www.sosfood.org

**Nebraska Sustainable Agriculture
Society**
www.nebsusag.org

Missouri Rural Crisis Center
www.morural.org

**Northwest Resistance Against
Genetic Engineering**
www.nwrage.org

Say No to GMOs! (Texas)
www.saynotogmos.org

*Genetic Engineering —
International*

Percy Schmeiser
www.percyschmeiser.com

ETC Group
www.etcgroup.org

Greenpeace International
*www.greenpeace.org/international/campaigns/ge-
netic-engineering*

Friends of the Earth International
www.foei.org

**GRAIN Genetic Resource Action
International**
www.grain.org

Network of Concerned Farmers
www.non-gm-farmers.com/index.asp

*Organic and Sustainable
Agriculture Organizations*

Organic Certifiers Directory
List maintained by the Organic Farming Research Foundation: *www.ofrf.org*

**California Certified Organic
Farmers**
1115 Mission St.
Santa Cruz, CA 95060
Phone: 831-423-2263
Toll Free: 888-423-2263
www.ccof.org

**Community Alliance with
Family Farmers**
P.O. Box 363
Davis, CA 95617
Phone: 530-756-8518
www.caff.org

**Community Food Security
Coalition**
P.O. Box 209
Venice, CA 90294
Phone: 310-822-5410
www.foodsecurity.org

Farm Aid
11 Ward St., Ste. 200
Somerville, MA 02143
Phone: 617-354-2922
Toll free: 800-FARM-AID
www.farmaid.org

**Food First/Institute for Food
& Development Policy**
398 60th St.
Oakland, CA 94618
Phone: 510-654-4400
www.foodfirst.org

**FoodRoutes: Where Does Your
Food Come From?**
37 East Durham Street
Philadelphia, PA 19119
Phone: 814-349-6000
www.foodroutes.org

Henry A. Wallace Center for Agricultural & Environmental Policy at Winrock International
2101 Riverfront Dr.
Little Rock, AR 72202
Phone: 501-280-3000
www.winrock.org

Independent Organic Inspectors Association
P.O. Box 6
Broadus, MT 59317
Phone: 406-436-2031
www.ioia.net

Leopold Center for Sustainable Agriculture
Iowa State University
209 Curtiss Hall
Ames, IA 50011
Phone: 515-294-3711
www.leopold.iastate.edu

Midwest Organic and Sustainable Education Service
P.O. Box 339
Spring Valley, WI 54767
Phone: 715-772-3153
www.mosesorganic.org

National Campaign for Sustainable Agriculture
P.O. Box 396
Pine Bush, NY 12566
Phone: 845-361-5201
www.sustainableagriculture.net

National Sustainable Agriculture Information Service
P.O. Box 3657
Fayetteville, AR 72702
Phone: 800-346-9140
www.attra.org

Northeast Organic Farming Association
c/o Bill Duesing
Box 135
Stevenson, CT 06491
Phone: 203-888-5146
www.nofa.org

Occidental Arts and Ecology Center
15290 Coleman Valley Rd.
Occidental, CA 95465
Phone: 707-874-1557
www.oaec.org

Organic Alliance
www.organicalliance.org

Organic Consumers Association
6771 South Silver Hill Dr.
Finland, MN 55603
Phone: 218-226-4164
www.organicconsumers.org

Organic Farming Research Foundation
P.O. Box 440
Santa Cruz, CA 95061
Phone: 831-426-6606
www.ofrf.org

Organic Trade Association
P.O. Box 547
Greenfield, MA 01302
Phone: 413-774-7511
www.ota.com

Rodale Institute
611 Siegfriedale Rd.
Kutztown, PA 19530
Farm: 610-683-1400
Bookstore: 800-832-6285
www.rodaleinstitute.org

Rural Advancement Foundation International USA
P.O. Box 640
7274 Pittsboro Elementary School Road
Pittsboro, NC 27312
Phone: 919-542-1396
www.rafiusa.org

Soil Association
Bristol House
40-56 Victoria St.
Bristol, BS1 6BY United Kingdom
Phone: 0117 314 5000
www.soilassociations.org

Sustainable Cotton Project
P.O. Box 363
Davis, CA 95617
Phone: 530-756-8518 ext.34
www.sustainablecotton.org

Western Association of Resource Councils
220 South 27th Street #B
Billings, MT 59101
Phone: 406-252-9672
www.worc.org

World-Wide Opportunities on Organic Farms (WWOOF)
P.O. Box 2675
Lewes BN7 1RB
England
United Kingdom
www.wwoof.org

USDA National Organic Program
USDA-AMS-TMP-NOP
Room 4008-South Building
1400 Independence Ave., S.W.
Washington, D.C. 20250-0020
Phone: 202-720-3252
www.ams.usda.gov/nop

Government Resources

U.S. House of Representatives
www.house.gov

U.S. Senate
www.senate.gov

Federal Agencies with Responsibility for Regulating Genetically Modified Crops and Foods

U.S. Food and Drug Administration (FDA)
www.cfsan.fda.gov/~lrd/biotechm.html

U.S. Department of Agriculture (USDA) *www.aphis.usda.gov/brs*

U.S. Environmental Protection Agency (EPA)
www.epa.gov/pesticides/biopesticides

U.S. Regulatory Agencies Unified Biotechnology Website
http://usbiotechreg.nbii.gov

GE crop field trials in the U.S.
www.nbiap.vt.edu/cfdocs/fieldtests1.cfm

GE field trials internationally
www.nbiap.vt.edu/cfdocs/globalfieldtests.cfm

FURTHER READING

APPENDIX 3B

Books

Aldridge, S. *The Thread of Life: The Story of Genes and Genetic Engineering*. New York: Cambridge University Press, 1996.

Anderson, Luke. *Genetic Engineering, Food, and Our Environment*. White River Junction, Vermont: Chelsea Green Publishing Co., 2000.

Bains, W. *Biotechnology from A to Z*. 2nd edition. Oxford: Oxford Press, 1998.

Becker, G.K., ed. *Changing Nature's Course: The Ethical Challenge of Biotechnology*. Hong Kong: Hong Kong University Press, 1996.

Borem, A., F. R. Santos, and D.E. Bowen. *Understanding Biotechnology*. Prentice Hall, 2003.

Charles, Daniel. *Lords of the Harvest: Biotech, Big Money, and the Future of Food*. Cambridge, MA: Perseus Publishing, 2001.

Cummins, Ronnie and Ben Lilliston. *Genetically Engineered Food: A Self Defense Guide for Consumers*. 2nd edition. New York: Marlowe and Company, 2004.

Davidson, Osha Gray. *Broken Heartland: The Rise of America's Rural Ghetto*. New York, NY: The Free Press, 1990.

Fowler, C. *Unnatural Selection: Technology, Politics and Plant Evolution*. Amsterdam: Gordon and Breach, 1994.

Fowler, C. and P. Mooney. *Shattering: Food, Politics, and the Loss of Genetic Diversity*. Tuscon: University of Arizona Press, 1990.

Fox, Michael. *Eating with Conscience: The Bioethics of Food*. NewSage Press, 1997.

Grace, E. *Biotechnology Unzipped: Promises and Realities*. Toronto: Trifolium Books, 1997.

Ho, Dr. Mae-Wan. *Genetic Engineering: Dream or Nightmare?* Bath, UK: Gateway Books, 1998.

Holdgrege, Craig. *Genetics and the Manipulation of Life: The Forgotten Factor of Context*. Hudson, NY: Lindisfarne Press, 1996.

Hubbard, R. and E. Wald. *Exploding the Gene Myth: How Genetic Information is Produced and Manipulated by Scientists, Physicians, Employers, Insurance Companies, Educators, and Law Enforcers*. Boston: Beacon Press, 1999.

Jack, Alex. *Imagine a World Without Monarch Butterflies*. One Peaceful World Press, 1999.

Keller, E.F. *Refiguring Life: Metaphors of Twentieth Century Biology*. New York: Columbia University Press, 1995.

Kimbrell, Andrew. *The Human Body Shop: The Engineering and Marketing of Life*. Harper Collins, 1993.

Kimbrell, Andrew. *Fatal Harvest: The Tragedy of Industrial Agriculture*. Island Press, 2002.

Kloppenburg, J.R., Jr. *First the Seed: The Political Economy of Plant Biotechnology*. Cambridge, MA: Cambridge University Press, 1988.

Kneen, B. *Farmageddon: Food and the Culture of Biotechnology*. New Society Publishers, 1999.

Lambrecht, Bill. *Dinner at the New Gene Café: How Genetic Engineering Is Changing What We Eat, How We Live, and the Global Politics of Food*. New York: St. Martin's Press, 2001.

Lappé, Marc and Brit Bailey. *Against the Grain: Biotechnology and the Corporate Takeover of Your Food*. Monroe, Maine: Common Courage Press, 1998.

Letourneau, Deborah K. and Beth Elpern Burrows, eds. *Genetically Engineered Organisms*. Boca Raton, FL: CRC Press, 2002.

Lycett, G.W. and D. Grierson. *Genetic Engineering of Crop Plants*. London: Butterworth, 1990.

Nelson, Gerald C., ed. *Genetically Engineered Organisms in Agriculture: Economics and Politics*. San Diego, Calif.: Academic Press, 2001.

Nestle, Marion. *Safe Food: Bacteria, Biotechnology, and Bioterrorism*. Berkeley, Calif.: University of California Press, 2003.

Nicholl, D.S.T. *An Introduction to Genetic Engineering*. New York: Cambridge University Press, 1994.

Rampton, Sheldon and John Stauber. *Trust Us We're Experts*. New York: Jeremy P. Tarcher/Putnam, 2001.

Rifkin, Jeremy. *The Biotech Century*. Tarcher/Putnam, 1998.

Robbins, John. *The Food Revolution: How Your Diet Can Help Save Your Life and Our World*. Berkeley, Calif.: Coneri Press, 2001.

Shiva, V. *Biopiracy: The Plunder of Nature and Knowledge*. Canada: South End Press, 1997.

Shiva, V. *Stolen Harvest*. Canada: South End Press, 2000.

Shiva, V. and I. Moser. *Biopolitics: A Feminist and Ecological Reader on Biotechnology*. London: Zed Books, 1995.

Smith, Jeffery M. *Seeds of Deception*. Fairfield, Iowa: Yes! Books, 2003.

Steinberg, M.L. and D.S. Cosloy. *Dictionary of Biotechnology and Genetic Engineering*. New York: Facts on File, 1994.

Tagliaferro, L. *Genetic Engineering: Progress or Peril?* Lerner Publications Co., 1997.

Teitel, Martin and Kimberly A. Wilson. *Genetically Engineered Food: Changing the Nature of Nature*. Rochester, Vermont: Park Street Press, 1999.

Ticciati, Robin and Laura. *Genetically Engineered Foods: Are They Safe? You Decide*. Los Angeles: Keats Publishing, 1998.

Tudge, C. *The Engineer in the Garden: Genes and Genetics: From the Idea of Heredity to the Creation of Life*. London: Jonathan Cape, 1993.

Turney, Jon. *Frankenstein's Footsteps: Science, Genetics and Popular Culture*. Yale University Press, 1998.

Scientific Reports

Arriola, Paul E. "Risks of Escape and Spread of Engineered Genes from Transgenic Crops to Wild Relatives." *AgBiotech News and Information* 9, 1997.

Arriola, Paul E. and Norman C. Ellstrand. "Crop-to-Weed Gene Flow in the Genus Sorghum (Poaceae): Spontaneous Interspecific Hybridization between Johnsongrass, Sorghum Halapense, and Crop Sorghum, S. Bicolor." *American Journal of Botany* 83 1996: 1153-60.

Benbrook, Charles M. "Genetically Engineered Crops and Pesticide Use in the U.S.: The First Nine Years." BioTech InfoNet Technical Paper #7, October 2004.

Bergelson, J.; C.B. Purrington; and G. Wichmann. "Promiscuity in Transgenic Plants."

Nature 395, 1998: 25.

Bernstein, Jonathan et al. "Clinical and Laboratory Investigation of Allergy to Genetically Modified Foods." Environmental Health Prospectus, vol. 111, 2003: 1114-21. British Medical Association. Genetically Modified Foods and Health: A Second Interim Statement. London: British Medical Association, 2004.

Brookes, Graham and Peter Barfoot. "Co-existence in North American Agriculture: Can GM Crops be Grown with Conventional and Organic Crops?" Dorcester, UK: Economics Ltd., 2004.

Chopra, S. et al. "rBST (Nutrilac) 'Gaps Analysis' Report." rBST Internal Review Team, Health Protection Branch, Health Canada, (April 21, 1998). The Crucible Group. "People, Plants, and Patients: The Impact of Intellectual Property on Trade, Plant Biodiversity, and Rural Society." Ottawa: International Development Research Centre, 1994.

de Visser, A.J.C. et al. "Crops of Uncertain Nature? Controversies and Knowledge Gaps Concerning Genetically Modified Crops: An Inventory." *Plant Research International*, Report 12, August 2000.

Devlin RH et al. "Population Effects of Growth Hormone Transgenic Coho Salmon Depend on Food Availability and Genotype by Environment Interactions," *Proc. Natl. Acad. Science USA* 101(25), 2004: 9303-08.

Ellstrand, Norman C. "When Transgenes Wander, Should We Worry?" *Plant Physiology* 125, 2001: 1543-1545.

Ellstrand N. "Dangerous Liaisons? When Cultivated Plants Mate with Their Wild Relatives," *The Johns Hopkins University Press* (2003).

Epstein, S.S. "Unlabeled Milk from Cows Treated with Biosynthetic Growth Hormones: A Case of Regulatory Abdication." *International Journal of Health Services* 26 (1996): 173-185.

Evaluation of Allergenicity of Genetically Modified Foods. Report of a Joint FAO/WHO Expert Consultation on Allergenicity of Foods Derived from Biotechnology. (January 22-25, 2001).

Ewen, Stanley W.B. and Arpad Puztai. "Effect of Diets Containing Genetically Modified Potatoes Expressing Galanthus Nivalis Lectin on Rat Small Intestine," *Lancet* 354, 1999.

Food and Agriculture Organization. The State of Food Insecurity in the World 2003: Monitoring Progress Toward the World Food Summit and Millennium Development Goals. FAO, Biotechnology Research, Italy (2003).

Food Ethics Council. Engineering Nutrition:

GM Crops for Global Justice. Brighton, UK: Food Ethics Council, 2003.

Fox, J.L. "Farmers Say Monsanto's Engineered Cotton Drops Bolls." *Nature Biotechnology* 15, 1997:1233.

Garrison, Jane. "'Agriscience Bus' Takes Teachers for a Ride." *Conscious Choice*, November 2003.

GM Science Review Panel. "GM Science Review (Second Report): An Open Review of the Science Relevant to GM Crops and Food Based on the Interests and Concerns of the Public." *The GM Science Review*, January 2004.

Gunning R.V. et al. "New Resistance Mechanism in Helicoverpa armigera Threatens Transgenic Crops Expressing Bacillus thuringiensis Cry1Ac toxin," *Appl. Environ. Microbiol.* 71(5), 2005: 2558-63.

Gurian-Sherman, Doug. "Holes in the Biotech Safety Net: FDA Policy Does Not Assure the Safety of Genetically Engineered Foods." Report from the Center for Science in the Public Interest (January 2003).

Hallman, W.K. et al. "Public Perceptions of Genetically Modified Foods: A National Study of American Knowledge and Opinion." Food Policy Institute publication number RR-103-004. Rutgers University, New Brunswick NJ (October 2003).

Harl, Neil E. et al. "The Starlink Situation." Iowa State University Extension Publications (April 2003).

Hilbeck, Angelika et al. "Toxicity of Bacillus thuringensis Cry1Ab Toxin to the Predator Chrysoperla carnea (Neuroptera: Chrysopiadae)," *Environmental Entomology* 27 1998: 1255-63.

Ho, Mae-Wan and Lim Li Ching. "The Case for a GM-Free Sustainable World." Report by the Institute of Science in Society & the Third World Network, Independent Science Panel (2003).

Ho, Mae-Wan and Angela Ryan. "Cauliflower Mosaic Viral Promoter-A Recipe for Disaster?" *Microbial Ecology in Health and Disease* no. 4, 1999.

Ho, Mae-Wan et al. "CaMV 35S Promoter Fragmentation Hotspot Confirmed, and It Is Active in Animals," *Microbial Ecology in Health and Disease*, vol. 13, 2000.

Inose, T. and K. Murata. "Enhanced Accumulation of Toxic Compound in Yeast Cells Having High Glycolytic Activity: A Case Study on the Safety of Genetically Engineered Yeast." *International Journal of Food Science and Technology* 30, 1995: 141-146.

James, Clive. "Preview: Global Status of Commercialized Transgenic Crops" (2003).

ISAAA Briefs no. 30. ISAAA: Ithaca, NY, 2003.

Jesse, Laura C.H. and John J. Obrycki. "Field Deposition of Bt Transgenic Corn Pollen: Lethal Effects on the Monarch Butterfly." *Oecologia* 125, 2000: 241.

Kareiva P., I.M. Parker, and M. Pascual. "Can We Use Experiments and Models in Predicting the Invasiveness of Genetically Engineered Organisms?" *Ecology* 77, 1999: 1670-75.

Kimura, T. et al. "Gastrointestinal Absorption of Recombinant Human Insulin-like Growth Factor-1 in Rats." *Journal of Pharmacology & Experimental Therapeutics*, 283, 1997: 611-618.

Kleter, G.A. and A.A.C.M. Peijnenburg. "Screening of Transgenic Proteins Expressed in Transgenic Food Crops for the Presence of Short Amino Acid Sequences Identical to Potential, IgE-binding Linear Epitopes of Allergens." *BMC Structural Biology*, vol. 2, 2002: 8-19.

Krimsky, S. and R. Wrubel. "Agricultural Biotechnology: An Environmental Outlook." Department of Urban and Environmental Policy, Tufts University, Medford, MA, 1993.

Lewis, W.J. et al. "A Total System Approach to Sustainable Pest Management," *PNAS* 94, 1997: 12,243-48.

Losey, J.E. et al. "Transgenic Pollen Harms Monarch Butterflies," *Nature* 399, 1999: 214.

Lui, Yong-Biao et al. "Development Time and Resistance to *Bt* Crops," *Nature* 400, 1999: 519.

Marvier, M, 2002, "Improving Risk Assessment for Non-target Safety of Transgenic Crops," *Ecol. Applica.* 12: 1119-24.

Mellon, M. and J. Rissler, "Gone to Seed: Transgenic Contaminants in the Traditional Seed Supply," Union of Concerned Scientists (2004).

Mellon, M., and J. Rissler. "Now or Never: Serious New Plans to Save a Natural Pest Control." Union of Concerned Scientists, 1998.

Mercer, D.K. et al. "Fate of Free DNA and Transformation of the Oral Bacterium Streptococcus Gordonii DL1 by Plasmid DNA in Human Saliva." *Applied and Environmental Microbiology* 65, 1999: 6-10.

Meyer, P., F. Linn, I. Heidmann et al. "Endogenous and Environmental Factors Influence 35 S Promoter Methylation of a Maize A1 Gene Construct in Transgenic Petunia and Its Colour Phenotype." *Molecular Genes and Genetics* 231, 1992: 345-352.

Meziani, Gundula and Hugh Warwick. "Seeds of Doubt: North American Farmers' Experiences of GM Crops." Report. Soil Association (September 2002).

Millstone, Erik et al. "Beyond 'Substantial Equivalence.'" *Nature* 401, 1999: 525-526.

Moeller, David R. "GMO Liability Threats for Farmers: Legal Issues Surrounding the Planting of Genetically Modified Crops." Institute for Agriculture and Trade Policy Report. Farmers' Legal Action Group, Inc., November 2001.

Muir, W. and R. Howard. "Possible Ecological Risks of Transgenic Organism Release when Transgenes Affect Mating Success: Sexual Selection and the Trojan Gene Hypothesis." *PNAS* 96, 1999: 13853-56.

National Research Council. "Biological Confinement of Genetically Engineered Organisms." *The National Academies Press*, Washington, D.C. (2004).

National Research Council. "Environmental Effects of Transgenic Plants; The Scope and Adequacy of Regulation." *The National Academies Press*, Washington, D.C (2004).

Nestle, Marion, Ph.D., M.P.H. "Allergies to Transgenic Foods—Questions of Policy." *The New England Journal of Medicine* 334, 1996.

Netherwood T., S.M. Martin-Orue, A.G. O'Donnell et al. "Assessing the Survival of Transgenic Plant DNA in the Human Gastrointestinal Tract." *Nat Biotechnol.* 22(2), 2004: 204-9.

Nordlee, Julie A., M.S. et al. "Identification of a Brazil-Nut Allergen in Transgenic Soybeans," *The New England Journal of Medicine* 334, 1996.

Obrycki, John J. et al. "Transgenic Insecticidal Corn: Beyond Insecticidal Toxicity to Ecological Complexity," *BioScience* 51, 2001: 354-355.

Pew Initiative on Food and Biotechnology. "Genetically Modified Crops in the United States." Fact Sheet, PEW Initiative on Food and Biotechnology, August 2004.

Prescott, V.E. et al. "Transgenic Expression of Bean Amylase Inhibitor in Peas Results in Altered Structure and Immunogenicity." J. Agric. Food Chem. 53, 2005: 9023-30.

Pusztai, Arpad. "Genetically Modified Foods: Are They a Risk to Human/Animal Health?" ActionBioscience.org, (June 2001).

Pryme, I.F., and R. Lembcke. "In Vivo Studies of Possible Health Consequences of Genetically Modified Food and Feed—With Particular Regard to Ingredients Consisting of Genetically Modified Plant Materials." *Nutrition and Health*, vol. 17, 2003: 1–8.

Quist, David and Ignacio H. Chapela, "Trans-

genic DNA Introgressed into Traditional Maize Landraces in Oaxaca, Mexico," *Nature* 414, 2001: 541-543.

Reddy, A.S. and T.L. Thomas. "Modification of Plant Lipid Composition: Expression of a cyanobacterial D6 –Desaturase Gene in Transgenic Plants." *Nature Biotechnology* vol. 14, 1996: 639-642.

Rissler, J. and M. Mellon. "Ecological Risks of Engineered Crops." MIT Press, Cambridge, MA, 1996.

Rissler, J. and M. Mellon. "Perils Amidst Promise: Ecological Risks of Transgenic Crops in a Global Market," Union of Concerned Scientists, Cambridge MA, 1993.

Saxena, Deepak et al. "Transgenic Plants: Insecticidal Toxin in Root Exudates from *Bt* Corn," *Nature* 402, 1999: 480.

Saxena, D., and G. Stotzky. "*Bt* Corn has a Higher Lignin Content than non-*Bt* Corn." *American J. Bot.* 88(9), 2001: 1704-06.

Schubert, David. "A Different Perspective on GM Food," *Nature Biotechnology*, vol. 20 2002: 969.

Snow, A.A., D.A. Andow, P. Gepts et al. "Genetically Engineered Organisms and the Environment: Current Status and Recommendations," ESA Position Paper. Ecological Society of America, Washington, D.C. (2004). *http://www.esa.org/pao/esaPositions/Papers/geo_position.htm*

Snow A.A. et al. "A *Bt* Transgene Reduces Herbivory and Enhances Fecundity in Wild Sunflowers," *Ecol. Applica.* 13(2), 2003: 279-286.

Somerville, C.R. and D. Bonetta, "Plants as Factories for Technical Materials." *Plant Physiology* 125, 2001: 168-171.

U.S. Department of Agriculture. Consumers and the Future of Biotech Foods in the U.S. Washington D.C.: USDA ERS, 2003.

VanGessel, M.J. "Glyphosate Resistant Horseweed from Delaware." *Weed Sci.* 49, 2001: 703-705.

Villar, Juan Lopez, ed. "Genetically Modified Crops: A Decade of Failure [1994-2004]." Friends of the Earth report, issue 105, 2004.

Villar, Juan Lopez, ed. "GMO Contamination Around the World." 2nd Edition Report for the Genetically Modified Organisms Programme, Friends of the Earth, August 2002.

Watrud, L. et al. "Evidence for Landscape-level, Pollen-mediated Gene Flow from Genetically Modified Creeping Bentgrass with CP4 EPSPS as a Marker." *Proc. Natl. Acad. Sci.* USA 101(40), 2004: 14533-38.

Williams, C.G. "Framing the Issues on Trans-

genic Forests." *Nature Biotechnology* 23(5), 2005: 530-532.

Wolfenbarger, L.L. and P.R. Phifer. "The Ecological Risks and Benefits of Genetically Engineered Plants." *Science* 290, 2000: 2088.

Wrubel, R.P., S. Krimsky et al. "Regulatory Oversight of Genetically Engineered Microorganisms: Has Regulation Inhibited Innovation?" *Journal of Environmental Management*, vol. 21 no. 4, 1997: 578.

Zhao, Jian-Zhou et al. "Development and Characterization of Diamondback Moth Resistance to Transgenic Broccoli Expressing High Levels of Cry1C," *Applied and Environmental Microbiology* 66, 2000: 3784-89.

Websites

Agribusiness Accountability Initiative: *www.agribusinessaccountability.org*

Genetically Engineered Organisms: Public Issues Education Project—Cornell University: *www.geo-pie.cornell.edu*

Iowa Rural Mental Health Initiative: *www.extension.iastate.edu/mentalhealth*

Mindfully.org: *www.mindfully.org/index.html*

University of Kentucky, Southeast Center for Agricultural Health and Injury Prevention: website on farmer suicide study: *www2.mc.uky.edu/Scahip/fmsuicide.htm*

Crop Choice—Alternative Farm News: *www.cropchoice.com*

ENDNOTES

Front Matter:

1: Jane Goodall, *Harvest for Hope: A Guide to Mindful Eating* (New York: Warner Books, 2005), 62.

Chapter 1:

1: Based on two opinion polls, both from Rutgers Food Policy Institute. The 2003 poll found that 94 percent of Americans want labeling; the 2004 poll found that 89 percent want labeling. Other opinion polls in the past four to five years have been in the same ballpark.
W.K. Hallman, W.C. Hebden, C.L. Cuite, H.L. Aquino, and J.T. Lang, "Americans and GM Food: Knowledge, Opinion and Interest in 2004," Food Policy Institute Report RR (2004): 1104-7.
W.K. Hallman. W. Hebden, H. Aquino, C. Cuite, and J. Lang, "Public Perceptions of Genetically Modified Foods: A National Study of American Knowledge and Opinion," Food Policy Institute Report RR (2003): 1003-4.

2: On the milk surplus, see: D.P. Blaney, J.J. Miller, and R.P. Stillman, "Dairy: Background for 1995 Farm Legislation" (USDA Agricultural Economics Report No. 705) (1995).

3: For a full discussion, see Doug Gurian-Sherman, "Holes in the Biotech Safety Net: FDA Policy Does Not Assure the Safety of Genetically Engineered Foods," Center for Science in the Public Interest, 2003, available at *http://www.cspinet.org/new/pdf/fda_report__final.pdf*

4: Ralph Nader, Foreword to *Genetically Engineered Food, Changing the Nature of Nature*. eds. Kimberly A. Wilson et al. (Vermont: Park Street Press, 2001), ix, x.

5: FDA, Freedom of Information Summary for POSILAC® (sterile sometribove zinc suspension) for Increasing Production of Marketable Milk in Lactating Dairy Cows, Sponsored by The Animal Sciences Division of Monsanto Company, available at *http://www.fda.gov/cvm/FOI/140872.pdf*

6: As reported in "Milk, Pregnancy, Cancer May Be Tied," Reuters, 10 September 2002. See also S. E. Hankinson, et al., "Circulating concentrations of insulin-like growth factor 1 and risk of breast cancer," *Lancet*, vol. 351, no. 9113, 1998: 1393-1396.

7: Adapted from "rBST (NUTRILAC) 'Gaps Analysis' Report" by the rBST Internal Review Team, Health Protection Branch, Health Canada (1998), available at *www.nfu.ca/gapsreport.html*

8: June M. Chan et al., "Plasma Insulin-like Growth Factor I and Prostate Cancer Risk: a Prospective Study." *Science*, vol. 279, 23 January 1998: 563-66. Also see Marian Burros, "A Hormone for Cows," *New York Times*, 9 November 2005.

9: Paul Kingsnorth, "Bovine Growth Hormones," *The Ecologist*, vol. 28, no. 5, September/October 1998. Also see FDA, Freedom of Information Summary for POSILAC® (sterile sometribove zinc suspension) for Increasing Production of Marketable Milk in Lactating Dairy Cows, Sponsored by The Animal Sciences Division of Monsanto Company, available at *www.fda.gov/cvm/FOI/140872.pdf*

10: GAO, "Recombinant Bovine Growth Hormone: FDA Approval Should Be Withheld until the Mastitis Issue Is Resolved." GAO/PEMD-92-26 (1992): 9.

11: For the EU see: "4. Summary and Conclusions" in the "Report on Public Health Aspects of the Use of Bovine Somatotrophin—15-16 March 1999" at *http://europa.eu.int/comm/food/fs/sc/scv/out19_en.html#_Toc446393145* For Canada, see: S. Chopra, M. Feeley, G. Lambert, et al., "rBST (Nutrilac): 'Gaps Analysis' Report" by the rBST Internal Review Team, Health Protec-

tion Branch, Health Canada, Canada (1998) at *http://www.nfu.ca/gapsreport. html#GAPS%20IN%20THE%20SCIENTIFIC%20DATA*

13: "Monsanto to Cut in Half Supply of Dairy Hormone: FDA's Tests of POSILAC in Australia Turn up Bacteria," *Baltimore Sun*, 14 February 2004.

14: Marian Burros, "A Hormone for Cows," *New York Times*, 9 November 2005.

15: Memo from FDA Division of Food Chemistry & Technology and FDA Division of Food Contaminants Chemistry to James Maryanski, Biotechnology Coordinator, "Points to Consider for Safety Evaluation of Genetically Modified Foods," 1 November 1991.

16: For instance, consider the CaMV 35S promoter, one of the most popular promoters in agricultural biotech. Research in cotton has shown, "After germination, varying levels of promoter activity were observed in all cell and tissue types in the hypocotyl, cotyledon, stem, leaf, petiole, and root." Sunilkumar et al. "Developmental and Tissue-Specific Expression of CaMV 35S Promoter in Cotton as Revealed by GFP." *Plant Mol Biol*. 50(3), 2003: 463-74.

17: Document from Dr. Louis J. Pribyl, "Comments on Biotechnology Draft Document," 6 March 1992.

18: Memorandum from Dr. Linda Kahl, FDA compliance officer, to Dr. James Maryanski, FDA's Biotechnology Coordinator, about the Federal Register document "Statement of Policy: Foods from Genetically Modified Plants," 8 January 1992.

19: Memorandum from Dr. Gerald B. Guest, Director of the Center for Veterinary Medicine, to Dr. James Maryanski, Biotechnology Coordinator. Subject: "Regulation of Transgenic Plants—FDA Draft Federal Register Notice on Food Biotechnology," 5 February 1992, available at *http://www.biointegrity. org/list.html*

20: Charles H.R.H., the Prince of Wales, "The Seeds of Disaster," *Daily Telegraph*, 8 June 1998, available at *http://www.princeofwales.gov.uk/speeches/agriculture_08061998.html*

21: Marion Nestle, Ph.D., MPH, "Allergies to Transgenic Foods – Questions of Policy." *New England Journal of Medicine* 334, no. 11, 1996.

22: J.A. Nordlee, S.L. Taylor, J.A. Townsend et al. "Identification of a Brazil Nut Allergen in Transgenic Soybeans," *New England Journal of Medicine* 334, 1996: 688-692.

23: V.E. Prescott et al., "Transgenic Expression of Bean—Amylase Inhibitor in Peas Results in Altered Structure and Immunogenicity," *Journal of Agricultural and Food Chemistry* vol. 53, issue 23, 2005: 9023-30.

24: For corn, soy, and cotton: USDA/NASS Acreage Report, 30 June 2005. Figures for canola are hard to come by. This figure is from Pew Initiative on Food and Biotechnology's "Factsheet: Genetically Modified Crops in the United States" (2001), available at *http://pewagbiotech.org/resources/factsheets/display.php3?FactsheetID=1*

25: "Guidance for Industry: Use of Antibiotic Resistance Marker Genes in Transgenic Plants," Draft released for comment on 4 September 1998. Food and Drug Administration, Center for Food Safety and Applied Nutrition, Center for Veterinary Medicine.

26: Ibid.

27: Courvalin, "Transgenic Plants and Antibiotics," *La Recherche* 309, 1998: 36-40.

28: The British Medical Association, which represents more that eighty percent of physicians in England, recommended that "there should be a ban on the use of antibiotic resistance marker genes in GM food, as the risk to human health from antibiotic resistance developing in micro-organisms is one of the major public health threats that will be faced in the 21st century," BMA Report, May 1999.

29: Memo from Dennis Ruggles, Experimental Design and Evaluation Branch, to Carl Johnson, Additives Evaluation Branch. "Statistical Analyses of Three 28-day Toxicity Studies in Charles River Crl: CD BR Rats Given a Transgenic Tomato," 7 June 1993.

30: A.N. Mayeno & G.J. Gleich, "Eosinophilia Myalgia Syndrome and Tryptophan Production: a Cautionary Tale." TIBTECH 12, 1994: 346-352.

31: Memo from FDA Division of Food Chemistry & Technology and FDA Division of Food Contaminants Chemistry to James Maryanski, Biotechnology Coordinator, "Points to Consider for Safety Evaluation of Genetically Modified Foods," 1 November 1991.

32: S.W. Ewen and A. Pusztai, "Effect of Diets Containing Genetically Modified Potatoes Expressing Galanthus Nivalis Lectin on Rat Small Intestine," *Lancet*, vol. 354, issue 9187, 1999: 1353-54.

33: Led by the London paper *The Independent*, 22 May 2005. Also see various articles accessible (under "Headlines") at *www.organicconsumers.org/monlink.html*

34: Memo from FDA Division of Food Chemistry & Technology and FDA Division of Food Contaminants Chemistry to James Maryanski, Biotechnology Coordinator, "Points to Consider for Safety Evaluation of Genetically Modified Foods," 1 November 1991.

35: Ibid.

36: Lappé et al., "Alterations in Clinically Important Phytoestrogens in Genetically Modified, Herbicide-Tolerant Soybeans." *Journal of Medicinal Food*, vol. 1, no. 4, 1999.

37: Iowa State University, "Research About 1% Linolenic Soybean Oil" (2004), available at *http://www.notrans.iastate.edu/research.html*

38: Andrew Kimbrell and Joseph Mendelson, Monsanto v. U.S. Farmers, 2005.

39: "Global Seed Industry Concentration – 2005," *The Action Group on Erosion, Technology, and Concentration*, issue 90, 2005.

40: David Barboza, "A Weed Killer Is a Block to Build On," *New York Times*, 2 August 2001.

41: See U.S. Dept. of Agriculture's website listing of "deregulated" GE crops at *http://www.aphis.usda.gov/brs/not_reg.html*

42: Much of this rejection is taking place due to the efforts of organizations like Oregon Physicians for Social Responsibility at *www.oregonpsr.org*. For a list of dairies that do not use rBGH, see the appendix.

43: See U.S. Dept. of Agriculture's website listing of "deregulated" GE crops at *http://www.aphis.usda.gov/brs/not_reg.html*

44: See Illinois Specialty Farm Products, "High Oleic Soybeans – Updated for 2003" at *http://web.aces.uiuc.edu/value/factsheets/soy/fact-oleic-soy.htm*

45: Yahoo business profile for Dow available at *http://biz.yahoo.com/ic/10/10471.html*

46: See U.S. Dept. of Agriculture's website listing of "deregulated" GE crops at *http://www.aphis.usda.gov/brs/not_reg.html*

47: See the "Syngenta AG" profile at *http://www.hoovers.com/syngenta/--ID__102664--/free-co-factsheet.xhtml*

48: Alison Pierce, "Bioscience Warfare," *SF Weekly*, 2 June 2004.

Chapter 2:

1: Andrew Kimbrell and Tracie Letterman, "The Catch with Seafood," Center for Food Safety (2005).

2: Jane Kay, "Frankenfish Spawn Controversy, Debate over Genetically Altered Salmon," *San Francisco Chronicle*, 29 April 2002, available at *www.sfgate.com*

3: Global Justice Ecology Project Press Release, "First Documentary on Genetically Engineered Trees Released," 10 November 2005, available at *http://globaljusticeecology.org*

4: W.M. Muir and R.D. Howard, "Possible Ecological Risks of Transgenic Organism Release When Transgenes Affect Mating Success: Sexual Selection and the Trojan Gene Hypothesis," Proc. Nat. Acad. Sci 96(24), 1999: 13853-56.

5: BBC News, "'Trojan' Gene Could Wipe Out Fish," 1 December 1999, available at *http://news.bbc.co.uk/1/hi/sci/tech/545504.stm*

6: Ibid.

7: Barry Commoner, "The Spurious Foundation of Genetic Engineering," *Harpers*, February 2002, available at *http://www.commondreams.org/views02/0209-01.htm*

8: T. Kent Kirk and John E. Carlson, *Biological Confinement of Genetically Engineered Organisms*, (Washington, D.C.: National Academies Press, 2004), available at *http://www.nap.edu/books/0309090857/html/*

9: L.S. Watrud, et al., "Evidence for Landscape-level, Pollen-mediated Gene Flow from Genetically Modified Creeping Bentgrass with CP4 EPSPS as a Marker," *Proc. Nat. Acad. Sci.* 101(40), 2004: 14533-38.

10: C. Hawes et al., "Responses of Plants and Invertebrate Trophic Groups to Contrasting Herbicide Regimes in the Farm Scale Evaluations of Genetically Modified Herbicide-Tolerant Crops," *Phil. Trans. R. Soc. Lond.* B, 358, 2003: 1899-1913. See also Maria Burke, "Managing GM Crops with Herbicides: Effects on Farmland Wildlife," Farmscale Evaluations Research Consortium and the Scientific Steering Committee, available at *http://www.defra.gov.uk/environment/gm/fse/results/fse-summary-05.pdf*

11: For U.S.: USDA, National Agricultural Statistics Service, Crop Acreage Report, 30 June 2005, available at *http://usda.mannlib.cornell.edu/reports/nassr/field/pcp-bba/acrg0605.pdf*. Internationally: C. James, "Highlights of ISAAA Briefs No. 34-2005: Global Status of Commercialized Biotech/GM Crops: 2005," 11 January 2006, available at *http://www.isaaa.org/kc/CBTNews/2006_Issues/Jan/Briefs_34_Highlights.pdf*

12: See two articles in *Weed Resistance Management*, vol. 8, no. 2, Winter 1996: Gressel, "Fewer Constraints than Proclaimed to the Evolution of Glyphosate-Resistant Weeds," and Sindel, "Glyphosate Resistance Discovered in Annual Ryegrass."

13: Leonard Gianessi, "Agricultural Biotechnology: Benefits of Transgenic Soybeans," National Center for Food and Agricultural Policy, April 2000: 62, 70-72, available at *http://www.ncfap.org/reports/biotech/rrsoybeanbenefits.pdf*.

14: Charles Benbrook, "Genetically Engineered Crops and Pesticide Use in the United States: The First Nine Years," Northwest Science and Environmental Policy Center, 25 October 2004.

15: David A. Bohan, et al., "Effects on Weed and Invertebrate Abundance and Diversity of Herbicide Management in Genetically Modified Herbicide-Tolerant Winter-sown Oilseed Rape," *Proc. R. Soc. B*, 2005: 272, 463–474, available at *http://www.journals.royalsoc.ac.uk/link.asp?id=xk8elc7n9j2au5tb*

16: R. Relyea, "The Impact of Insecticides and Herbicides on the Biodiversity and Productivity of Aquatic Communities," *Ecological Applications*, 15(2), 2005: 618-627.

17: M.J. VanGessel, "Glyphosate Resistant Horseweed from Delaware," *Weed Sci.* 49, 2001: 703-705.

18: Iowa State University, Weed Science Department, "Preserving the Value of Glyphosate," joint statement released by 12 Midwestern weed scientists, 20 February, 2004, available at *http://www.weeds.iastate.edu/mgmt/2004/preserving.shtml*

19: For instance, see Monsanto's own website on weed resistance management at *http://www.weedresistancemanagement.com*. The company recommends that farmers "[i]ncorporate other herbicides and cultural practices as part of Roundup Ready® cropping systems where appropriate."

20: R.M. Goodman and N. Newell, "Genetic Engineering of Plants for Herbicide Resistance: Status and Prospects," *Engineered Organisms in the Environment: Scientific Issues*, eds. H. O. Halvorson, D. Pramer and M. Rogul, (Washington D.C.: American Society for Microbiology, 1985): 47-53, available at *http://www.sci.uidaho.edu/biosci/lecture/Top/Bio%20411%20s%2005/When%20Transgenes%20Wander_Ellstrand.pdf*

21: National Research Council, Board on Agriculture and Natural Resources,

"Environmental Effects of Transgenic Plants: The Scope and Adequacy of Regulation," *National Academy Press*, 2002.

22: Hall et al., "Pollen Flow between Herbicide-Resistant Brassica napus is the Cause of Multiple-Resistant B. napus Volunteers," *Weed Science*: vol. 48, no. 6, 2000: 688-694.

23: The Royal Society of Canada, "Elements of Precaution: Recommendation for the Regulation of Food Biotechnology in Canada," January 2001: 122-123.

24: Mike J. Wilkinson, Luisa J. Elliott, Joël Allainguillaume et al., "Hybridization Between Brassica napus and B. rapa on a National Scale in the United Kingdom," *Science*, vol. 302, issue 5644, 2003: 457-459, available at *http://www.sciencemag.org/cgi/content/full/302/5644/457*. Also see "Crops that Keep Their Genes to Themselves," *Nature Biotechnology*, April 1999: 390-392, 330-331, available at *http://www.nature.com/nbt/press_release/nbt0499.html*

25: Michael Pollan, *The Botany of Desire: A Plant's Eye View of the World* (New York: Random House, 2002), 197.

26: Charles Benbrook, "Genetically Engineered Crops and Pesticide Use in the United States: The First Nine Years," BioTech InfoNet, Technical Paper Number 7, October 2004: 53, available at *http://www.biotech-info.net/technicalpaper7.html*

27: Leonard Gianessi, "Agricultural Biotechnology: Benefits of Transgenic Soybeans," National Center for Food and Agricultural Policy, April 2000: 62, 70-72, available at *http://www.ncfap.org/reports/biotech/rrsoybeanbenefits.pdf*.

28: Ibid.

29: Charles M. Benbrook, "Troubled Times Amid Commercial Success for Roundup Ready Soybeans," Northwest Science and Environmental Policy Center, 3 May 2001, available at *http://www.biotech-info.net/troubledtimes.html*

30: Stephen J. Toth, ed. "Plant Bugs and Stink Bugs on Cotton," *North Carolina Pest News*, vol. 19, no. 13, 2003.

31: Oregon Potato Commission, "Evaluation of Alternative Insecticides to Replace those at Risk from FQPA," Progress Report to the Agricultural Research Foundation, (1999-2000): 13.

32: Rocco Moschetti, "Microbial Insecticide Profile: Bacillus thuringiensis," IPM of Alaska (2002), available at *http://www.ipmofalaska.com/files/BTprofile.html*

33: Lewis et al., "A Total System Approach to Sustainable Pest Management." *Proc. Nat. Acad. Sci.*, vol. 94 (1997): 12243-12248.

34: John W. Van Duyn and Wayne Modlin, "Corn Insect Management with Transgenic Bt Corn in North Carolina," North Carolina State University, available at *http://www.ces.ncsu.edu/plymouth/pubs/btcorn99.html*. In reference to two common kinds of Bt corn, they write, "These [Bt] gene events express a high toxin concentration during the entire season…"

35: Deepak Saxena et al., "Transgenic Plants: Insecticidal Toxin in Root Exudates From Bt Corn," *Nature*, 402, 1999: 480. Also see J.E. Losey, L.S. Rayor, and M.E. Carter, "Transgenic Pollen Harms Monarch Larvae," *Nature* 399, 1999: 214 and A. Hilbeck, M. Baunigartner, P.M. Fried, and F. Bigler, "Effects of Transgenic Bacillus thuringiensis Corn-fed Prey on Mortality and Development Time of Immature Chysoperla carnea (Neuroptera: Chrysopidae)," *Environmental Entomology* 27(2), 1998: 480-487.

36: J.E. Losey, L.S. Rayor, and M.E. Carter, "Transgenic Pollen Harms Monarch Larvae," *Nature* 399, 1999: 214.

37: Hellmich et al., "Monarch Sensitivity to Bacillus thuringiensis-Purified Proteins and Pollen." *PNAS* 98, 2001: 11925-30; Oberhauser et al., "Temporal and Spatial Overlap between Monarch Larvae and Corn Pollen," *PNAS* 98, 2001: 11913-18; and M.K. Sears, et al., "Impact of *Bt* Corn Pollen on Monarch Butterfly Populations: A Risk Assessment," *PNAS* 98, 2001: 11937-42.

38: Zangerl et al., "Effects of Exposure to Event 176 Bacillus thuringiensis Corn Pollen on Monarch and Black Swallowtail Caterpillars under Field Conditions," *Proc. Natl. Acad. Sci.* 98, 2001: 11908-12.

39: Margaret Mellon and Jane Rissler, "Environmental Effects of Genetically Modified Food Crops," Recent Experiences (2003), Union of Concerned Scientists, available at *http://www.ucsusa.org/food_and_environment/biotechnology/page.cfm?pageID=1219*. Note: Syngenta, the company that created Event 176, allowed the product's pesticide registration to expire in 2001. EPA permitted the company to sell existing stocks of Event 176 corn through the 2003 growing season. (EPA, Biopesticides Registration Action Document, Bt Plant Incorporated Protectants, 15 October 2001, available at *http://www.epa.gov/oppbppd1/biopesticides/pips/bt_brad2/1-overview.pdf*)

40: A. Hilbeck, M. Baunigartner, P.M. Fried, and F. Bigler, "Effects of Transgenic Bacillus thuringiensis Corn-fed Prey on Mortality and Development Time of Immature Chysoperla carnea (Neuroptera: Chrysopidae)." *Environmental Entomology* 27 (2), 1998: 480-487.

41: J.Z. Zhao, H.L. Collins, and J.D. Tang et al., "Development and Characterization of Diamondback Moth Resistance to Transgenic Broccoli Expressing High Levels of Cry1C," *Applied Environmental Microbiology* 66, 2000: 3784-89.

42: R.V. Gunning et al., "New Resistance Mechanism in Helicoverpa armigera Threatens Transgenic Crops Expressing Bacillus thuringiensis Cry1AC toxin," *Appl. Environ. Microbiol.* 71(5), 2005: 2558-63.

43: E. Walz, "Third Biennial National Organic Farmers' Survey," Organic Farming Research Foundation, (2005), available at *http://www.ofrf.org/publications/survey/Final.Results.Third.NOF.Survey.pdf*

44: Rick Weiss, "Human Cloning Bid Stirs Experts' Anger; Problems in Animal Cases Noted," *The Washington Post*, 7 March 2001.

45: "Duplicate Dinner," *New Scientist*, 19 May 2001.

46: Melissa Schorr, "Geneticists Warn Of Human Cloning Dangers," *Reuters Health*, 29 March 2001.

47: Renard et al., "Lymphoid Hypoplasia and Somatic Cloning," *Lancet*, vol. 353, no. 9163, 1 May 1999; also, "Cloning May Cause Long Lasting Health Problems," *Lancet* press release, 1 May 1999.

48: John G. Vandenbergh, National Research Council, "Animal Biotechnology: Science-Based Concerns," Public Briefing, 21 August 2002, available at *http://www4.nationalacademies.org/news.nsf/isbn/s0309084393?OpenDocument*

49: The Royal Society of Canada, "Elements of Precaution: Recommendations for the Regulation of Food Biotechnology in Canada," Ottawa, The Royal Society of Canada for Health Canada, Canadian Food Inspection Agency, and Environment Canada. The Standing Senate Committee (2001): 87.

Chapter 3:

1: P. Gunderson, B. Donner, R. Nashold et al., "The Epidemiology of Suicide Among Farm Residents or Workers in Five North-central States, 1980-1988," Farm Injuries: A Public Health Approach, *American Journal of Preventative Medicine* 9, 1993: 26-32.

2: Wangari Maathai, "The Linkage Between Patenting of Life Forms, Genetic Engineering and Food Insecurity," The Green Belt Movement, 28 May 1998, available at *http://www.genet-info.org/-documents/AfricaGMOsPatents.pdf*

3: See Soil Association, "Seeds of Doubt: North American Farmers' Experiences of GM Crops" (2003): 28.

4: Ibid., Section 10: National Farm Economy.

5: Ibid., Section 10: National Farm Economy.

6: Alan Sipress and Marc Kaufman, "U.S. Challenges E.U. Biotech Food Standards," *Washington Post*, 26 August 2001.

7: Ramsay, Thompson, and Squire, "Quantifying Landscape-scale Gene Flow in Oilseed Rape." Report of U.K. Department for Environment, Food, and Rural Affairs, (2003), available at *http://www.defra.gov.uk/environment/gm/research/pdf/epg_rg0216.pdf*

8: Squire, Begg, and Askew, "Final Report of the DEFRA Project: Consequences for Agriculture of the Introduction of Genetically Modified Crops, RG0114," Report of U.K. Department of Environment, Food, and Rural

Affairs, (2003), available at *http://www.defra.gov.uk/environment/gm/research/pdf/epg_rg0114.pdf*

9: Watrud et al., "Evidence for Landscape-level, Pollen-mediated Gene Flow from Genetically Modified Creeping Bentgrass with CP4 EPSPS as a Marker," *PNAS* 101(40), 2004: 14533-38.

10: Union of Concerned Scientists, "Gone to Seed: Transgenic Contaminants in the Traditional Seed Supply," 2004.

11: For instance, see the European Cultivated Potato Database at *http://www.europotato.org/menu.php* and the Centro Internacional de la Papa at *http://www.cipotato.org/potato/potato.htm*

12: Biing-Hwan Lin et al., "Fast Food Growth Boosts Frozen Potato Consumption," *Food Review*, vol. 24, no. 1, 2001: 38-46.

13: FAO, "Biodiversity for Food and Agriculture: Crop Genetic Resources," February 1998, available at *http://www.fao.org/WAICENT/FAOINFO/SUSTDEV/EPdirect/EPre0040.htm*

14: See SeedQuest analysis based on USDA data, March 2003, available at *http://www.seedquest.com/statistics/usa/publicseedtradereports/2003/march.htm*

15: For instance, in June 2000, the world's largest vegetable seed company announced it would eliminate 2,000 varieties, or 25 percent of its entire product line. See Seminis press release, "Seminis Announces Global Restructuring and Optimization Plan," 28 June 2000, available at *http://seminis.com/news/news_2000/PR_2000_June28.html*

16: FAO, "Dimensions of Need: An Atlas of Food and Agriculture," Rome, 1995, available at *http://www.fao.org/documents/show_cdr.asp?url_file=/docrep/U8480E/U8480E00.htm*

17: Ibid.

18: This account based on the following sources: *www.percyschmeiser.com*; Rich Weiss, "Seeds of Discord: Monsanto's Seed Police Raise Alarm on Farmers' Rights, Rural Tradition," *Washington Post*, 3 February 1999; Daniel Charles, *Lords of the Harvest: Biotech, Big Money and the Future of Food* (New York: Perseus Publishing, 2001): 188-189.

19: See Supreme Court of Canada decision in Monsanto Canada Inc. v. Schmeiser (2004), available at *http://www.lexum.umontreal.ca/csc-scc/en/pub/2004/vol1/html/2004scr1_0902.html*

20: Elizabeth A. Castelli, "How?: What Can We Do about the State of the World? - A Panel of Activists" Adapted from the audio. The Scholar & Feminist Online, vol. 2, issue 2 (2004). *http://www.barnard.columbia.edu/sfonline/reverb/castell2.htm*

21: Based on DuPont company website "Meet the Executives," *http://www2.dupont.com/Our_Company/en_US/executives/fisher.html*; "A Matter of Trust: How the Revolving Door Undermines Public Confidence in Government – and What To Do About It," Revolving Door Working Group, October 2005, available at *http://www.revolvingdoor.info/docs/matter-of-trust_final-full.pdf*; Al Kamen, "Clinton Assistant Going Private," *Washington Post*, 21 April 1997.

22: Center for Food Safety, Monsanto v. U.S. Farmers, 2005. This information was compiled from public court records.

23: See Peter Shinkle, "Monsanto Reaps Some Anger with Hard Line on Reusing Seed," *St. Louis Post-Dispatch*, 19 May 2003. Although Monsanto has since denied that this is true, Monsanto's own Seed Piracy Update from 2003 states, "About $10 million per year is invested in protecting seed trait value..." by which they mean investigating and suing farmers.

24: Monsanto Co., "Monsanto Releases Seed Piracy Case Settlement Details," press release, 29 Sept 1998.

25: Rich Weiss, "Seeds of Discord: Monsanto's Gene Police Raise Alarm on Farmer's Rights, Rural Tradition," *Washington Post*, 3 February 1999.

26: In its 2004 "Seed Piracy Update," Monsanto claimed, "Nearly 600 new seed piracy matters were opened in 2003." Also an *Omaha World-Herald* article from November 2004 stated that Monsanto would investigate 500 farmers in 2004 "as it does every year." See "Bean Detectives Visit Nebraskan," 7 November 2004.

27: USDA Economic Research Service, Agricultural Biotechnology Intellectual Property. "This database identifies and describes U.S. utility patents on inventions in biotechnology and other biological processes—with issue dates between 1976 and 2000—that are used in food and agriculture," available at *http://www.ers.usda.gov/Data/AgBiotechIP/Data/Table10_Top100USNonUSSummarySubs.html*

28: Based on Center for Food Safety research using Public Access to Court Electronic Records (PACER). Research through the end of 2004 is documented in the CFS report, Monsanto v. U.S. Farmers, available at *www.centerforfoodsafety.org*

29: Monsanto Co., "Seed Piracy Update," 2004.

30: Center for Food Safety, Monsanto v. U.S. Farmers, 2005. This information was compiled from public court records.

31: Ibid.

32: Ibid.

33: Rose Marie Berger, "Web Exclusive: Wendell Berry interview complete text," *Sojourners Magazine*, vol. 33, no. 7, 2004, available at *http://www.sojo.net/index.cfm?action=magazine.article&issue=soj0407&article=040710x*

34: USDA, Agricultural Research Service, "Why USDA's Technology Protection System (aka 'Terminator') Benefits Agriculture," available at *http://www.ars.usda.gov/is/br/tps*

Chapter 4:

1: For instance, China, Japan, the EU, Australia, Russia, and Mexico all have labeling requirements. See the Center for Food Safety's "Genetically Engineered Crops and Foods: Worldwide Regulation and Prohibition" (October 2005).

2: For corn, soy, and cotton: USDA/NASS Acreage report, 30 June 2005. Figures for canola are hard to come by. This figure is cited in the Pew Initiative on Food and Biotechnology's "Factsheet: Genetically Modified Crops in the United States" (2001), available at *http://pewagbiotech.org/resources/factsheets/display.php3?FactsheetID=1*

3: USDA National Organic Program Standards available at *http://www.ams.usda.gov/nop/NOP/standards.html*

4: International Federation of Produce Coding "FAQs," available at *http://www.plucodes.com/plucodesfaq.asp*.

5: Hawaii Agricultural Statistics Service, Papaya Acreage Survey Results, August 2002, available at *http://www.nass.usda.gov/hi/fruit/annpap.htm*

6: Cornell Cooperative Extension's Genetically Engineered Organisms, Public Issues Education Project, "GE Foods in the Marketplace," (2002), available at *http://www.geo-pie.cornell.edu/educators/downloads/fs1_foods.pdf*

7: Wendell Berry, "The Pleasures of Eating" in *What Are People For?* (San Francisco: North Point Press, 1990)

8: Marian Burros, "Chefs Join Effort to Label Genetically Engineered Food," *New York Times*, 9 December 1998.

9: Maine Department of Agriculture, Food & Rural Resources, Division of Quality Assurance and Regulations. "Chapter 136: Official State of Maine Grades and Standards for Milk and Milk Products for Use with the State of Maine Quality Trademark," available at *ftp://ftp.state.me.us/pub/sos/cec/rcn/apa/01/001/001c136.doc*

10: USDA/NASS Acreage report, 30 June 2005.

11: USDA/Food Safety and Inspection Service (FSIS) "Meat and Poultry Labeling Terms," available at *www.fsis.usda.gov/Frame/FrameRedirect.asp?main=/oa/pubs/lablterm.htm*. Updated August 2003.

12: Alice Waters. "The Ethics of Eating: Why Environmentalism Starts at the Breakfast Table," *The Fatal Harvest Reader: The Tragedy of Industrial Agriculture,* ed.

Andrew Kimbrell, (Washington: Island Press, 2002), 283.

13: Robin Lee Allen, "New York Chefs Speak out Against Genetic Engineering." *Nation's Restaurant News*, 15 June 1992.

14: Center for Food Safety, "Genetically Engineered Crops and Foods: Worldwide Regulation and Prohibition." February 2006, available at *http://www.centerforfoodsafety.org/geneticall5.cfm*

15: Marian Burros, "Chefs Join Effort to Label Genetically Engineered Food," *New York Times*, 9 December 1998.

16: USDA/Food Safety and Inspection Service (FSIS) "Meat and Poultry Labeling Terms" available at *www.fsis.usda.gov/Frame/FrameRedirect.asp?main=/oa/pubs/lablterm.htm*. Updated August 2003.

17: Statement of the U.S. Popcorn Board, available at *http://www.popcorn.org/frames.cfm?main=about*. The Popcorn Board is a non-profit organization funded by U.S. popcorn processors. The Popcorn Board is also a national commodity promotion and research program.

18: "Solutions to GM Pollen Drift Face Patent, Funding Obstacles." *Non-GMO Report*, July 2005.

19: Sam Hananel, "Anheuser-Busch Threatens Mo. Rice Boycott," Associated Press, 12 April 2005.

20: *Sacramento Business Journal*, 17 April 1998.

Chapter 5:

1: Mikhail Gorbachev, "The Third Pillar of Sustainable Development," Preface to *The Earth Charter in Action: Toward a Sustainable World*. (Amsterdam: KIT Publishers BV, 2005).

2: Dennis Kucinich, "Summary of Genetically Engineered Food Legislation," available at *http://kucinich.house.gov/UploadedFiles/genetic_longsummary.pdf*

3: USDA Economic Research Service, "Organic Production 1992-2003," available at *http://www.ers.usda.gov/Data/organic/*

4: USDA Economic Research Service, "Organic Food Industry Taps Growing American Market," *Agricultural Outlook*, October 2002, available at *http://www.ers.usda.gov/publications/agoutlook/oct2002/ao295b.pdf*

5: Use of genetically engineered seed is an "excluded method" in organic agriculture. For the full National Organic Standards, see USDA National Organic Program at *http://www.ams.usda.gov/nop/indexIE.htm*

6: Table based on "Consumer Expenditures in 2002: Report 974," U.S. Dept. of Labor, Bureau of Labor Statistics (2004), available at *http://stats.bls.gov/cex/csxann02.pdf*

7: Vandana Shiva, "Biotech Wars: Food Freedom vs. Food Slavery," *ZNet Daily Commentaries*, 23 June 2003, available at *http://www.zmag.org/sustainers/content/2003-06/23shiva.cfm*

8: Rebecca Spector, "Fully Integrated Food Systems: Regaining Connections between Farmers and Consumers," *The Fatal Harvest Reader: The Tragedy of Industrial Agriculture*, ed. Andrew Kimbrell (Washington, D.C.: Island Press, 2002): 288-294.

9: Ibid.

10: Diane Conners, "Hunger Grows for Locally Grown Food," Great Lakes Bulletin News Service, 30 March 2005, available at *http://mlui.org/growthmanagement/fullarticle.asp?fileid=16831*

11: Message of His Holiness Pope John Paul II for the Celebration of the World Day of Peace, 1 January 1990. "Peace with God the Creator, Peace with All of Creation," available at *http://www.vatican.va/holy_father/john_paul_ii/messages/peace/documents/hf_jp-ii_mes_19891208_xxiii-world-day-for-peace_en.html*

12: The O'Mama Report, The Organic Trade Association, 5 January 2005.

13: World Council of Churches & World Association for Christian Communication, "Transforming Life: Genetics, Agriculture and Human Life," 3-54. The

policy was approved in February 2006.

14: Carol Ness, "Fighting for the Future of Food: Deborah Koons Garcia's Film Documents How Genetically Engineered Foods Slipped into our Supply," *San Francisco Chronicle*, 7 November 2004, available at *http://sfgate.com/cgi-bin/article.cgi?file=/c/a/2004/11/07/LVG709K7MV1.DTL*

15: Ann Bailey, "Boon or Bust? Opinion Divided over Whether Agragen Project Will Be a Help or Hindrance to Flax Industry" *Agweek*, 9 May 2005.

16: Associated Press, 15 June 2005.

17: Ann Bailey, "Boon or Bust? Opinion Divided over Whether Agragen Project Will Be a Help or Hindrance to Flax Industry" *Agweek*, 9 May 2005.

18: Full text of Boxer's letter available at *http://www.progress.org/archive/gene41.htm*

Appendices

1: Many of the companies listed here were found on a great resource on rBGH-free food complied by Mothers & Others and Rural Vermont: *www.checnet.org/healthehouse/pdf/milkchart.pdf*.

2: Alta Dena Dairy, "Our farmers do not treat their cows with rBST, Recombinant Bovine Somatotropin, a genetically engineered hormone." "Alta Dena Dairy Products." *www.altadenadairy.com/addProducts.asp*. Phone: 925/757-9209.

3: Brown Cow Farm, "At Brown Cow, we will not knowingly purchase or use milk from cows treated with the artificial growth hormone." "Crafted With Care." *www.browncowfarm.com/CraftedWithCare/index.cfm*. Phone: 925-757-9209.

4: Lifetime Dairy, Statement e-mailed 9/23/04, "Our suppliers have assured us that the milk used to manufacture Lifetime® Cheeses is rBGH/rBST-free." Phone: 831-899-5040.

5: Stonyfield Farms, "We only use premium milk from farmers who have pledged not to use the synthetic bovine growth hormone, rBGH." "About Us" *www.stonyfield.com/AboutUs*. Phone: 603-437-5050.

6: Ben & Jerry's Ice Cream website, "All of our milk and cream comes from a cooperative of Vermont dairy farmers who have pledged not to treat their cows with rBGH." "Support Home Page." *benjerry.custhelp.com/cgi-bin/benjerry.cfg/php/enduser/std_alp.php?p_sid=BfyZjtVg&p_lva=&p_sp=&p_li=*. Phone: 802-846-1500.

7: Franklin Foods, "All of our products still start with fresh milk from Vermont farms where cows are not treated with growth-stimulating hormones (rBGH)." "About Us" *www.franklinfoods.com/about.shtml*. Phone: 802-933-4338.

8: Crowley Cheese of Vermont, "Cheese Shop" Confirmed rBGH-free at: *www.crowleycheese-vermont.com/store/*. Phone: 802-259-2210.

9: Grafton Village Cheese Company, "Components" Confirmed rBGH-free at: *www.graftonvillagecheese.com/cheeseco/making/components.html*. Phone: 802/843-2221.

10: Great Hill Dairy, Customer Service representative, "There is no rBST in the milk. We have signed affidavits from all the farmers," 10/26/05. Phone: 508-748-2208.

11: Alpenrose Dairy, "Alpenrose Dairy Goes rBGH-free" announcement. Phone: 503-244-1133.

12: Clover Stornetta Dairy, "Our Philosophy on rBGH" Confirmed rBGH-free at: *www.clo-the-cow.com/philosophy.html*. Phone: 800-237-3315.

13: Joseph Farms Cheese, "We are the first cheese producer nationwide to be granted governmental approval to label our cheese 'No Artificial Hormones' (that means no rBGH/rBST either), and we're vegetarian too." From website, 10/25/05: *http://www.josephfarms.com/*. Phone: 209-394-7984.

14: Tillamook Cheese, "Since April 1, 2005, all TCCA members and contract milk suppliers for our cheese production are in compliance certifying that milk for cheese production delivered to our facilities in Boardman, OR and Tillamook, OR is from cows not supplemented with rBST... Our first priority has been the milk used in our cheese because cheese makes up 85 percent of our sales. Milk for some of our other dairy products comes from other suppliers. We are in the process of contacting those milk suppliers seeking to implement the same policy for all Tillamook dairy products. However, full implementation will take some time."

15: Berkeley Farms, "At Berkeley Farms, we make sure our milk is certified rBST hormone-free," "Get to Know Your Milk," *www.berkeleyfarms.com/get2. htm*. Phone: 510-265-8600.

16: Wilcox Family Farms, "Wilcox Family Farms' no artificial growth hormone rBST dairy line is available in a variety of locations." "Natural Products," *www.wilcoxfarms.com/rbst.html*, accessed 10/26/05.

17: Sunshine Dairy, "We are allied with Dairy Farmers that practice sustainable farming and are rBST free," "rBST Info," *http://www.sunshinedairyfoods. com/pages/rbst-d.html*, accessed 10/26/05.

18: Westby Creamery, "Our Products," *www.westbycreamery.com/products*. Phone: 800-492-9282.

19: Chippewa Valley Cheese, "Who We Are" confirmed rBGH-free at: *www. chippewavalleycheese.com/newwhoweare2.html*. Phone: 715-597-2366.

20: Promised Land Dairy website, "Our Products" confirmed rBGH-free at: *www.promisedlanddairy.com/Ourpercent20Products.html*. Phone: 210-533-9151.

21: Erivan Dairy Yogurt. "We use no hormone treatments whatsoever. We have one farm so we can monitor these things." Paul Fereshetian, farm manager. 10/27/05. Phone: 215-887-2009.

22: Crescent Creameries. Customer Service representative, "We have signed affidavits from farmers stating that they do not use rBST on their cows." 10/26/05. Phone: 800-221-6455.

23: Vermont Cheese Council, "Blythedale Farm" confirmed rBGH-free at: *www.vtcheese.com/vtcheese/blythedale/blythedale.htm*. Phone: 802-439-6575.

24: Erivan Dairy Yogurt. "We use no hormone treatments whatsoever. We have one farm so we can monitor these things." Paul Fereshetian, farm manager, 10/27/05. Phone: 215-887-2009.

25: Derle Farms, "We only use suppliers that don't use rBST. Have it in writing." Consumer representative Mr. Rabin. Phone: 718-257-2040.

26: Farmland Dairies, "Farmland Dairies farmers have pledged in writing that they will not use rBST on their cows." *http://www.farmlanddairies.com/rBGHpercent20new.htm*, accessed 10/27/05.

27: Wilcox Family Farms, "Wilcox Family Farms' no artificial growth hormone rBST dairy line is available in a variety of locations." "Natural Products," *http://www.wilcoxfarms.com/rbst.html*, accessed 10/26/05.

28: Oakhurst Dairy website, "Artificial Growth Hormone" confirmed rBGH-free at: *www.oakhurstdairy.com/bovine.html*.

29: Land O'Lakes, "Land O'Lakes, Inc. believes our dairy producers have the right to produce safe, high-quality milk using any approved and available technology. Currently, a small percentage of our farmer-members choose to use rBST in the management of their herds." Customer Service, 9/30/04.

30: Kemp, "Kemps 'Select' milk is the only product that we can guarantee comes from cows that are not treated with the bovine growth hormone." Customer Service, 9/30/04.

31: Sorrento, "We have no way of knowing which of our milk is treated [with rBST] and which is not, so we don't make a statement." Qualtity Department Director Tony Lardo, 10/27/05.

32: Yoplait, "It's certainly possible that some of our products may contain ingredients that have been improved through biotechnology." Jenny Path, General Mills Consumer Services, 11/7/05.

33: Colombo, "It's certainly possible that some of our products may contain ingredients that have been improved through biotechnology." Jenny Path, General Mills Consumer Services, 11/7/05.

34: Parmalat, "We cannot claim that the milk in Parmalat is free of genetically engineered hormones. We have not yet reached 100 percent satisfaction from our dairy farmers where these products come from—they are produced in Michigan." Customer Service representative, 11/1/05.

35: Dannon, Consumer Response representative Cindy Bauman, "We [Dannon] agree that using new production technologies can help our food production system as long as these new technologies have been approved as safe by the FDA." 9/21/04.

36: Silk website, "FAQs," "All soybeans used are organic and biotech-free." *www.silkissoy.com/index.php?id=17&cid=3#43*.

37: EdenSoy website, "Since 1993 Eden's Purchasing Department, with their suppliers, has protected their patrons and does everything possible to make sure their food is free of GEOs." "GEO Stance," *www.edenfoods.com/issues_geo. html*.

38: Imagine Foods, "Imagine Foods does not use ingredients that were produced using biotechnology." "Info Center," *www.imaginefoods.com/pages/info/gmo.php*.

39: Tofutti website, "FAQs," "All of our products use non-GMO soy protein. In addition, if available, we use other non-GMO ingredients." *www.tofutti.com*.

40: VitaSoy, "FAQs," "Vitasoy USA uses only non-GMO ingredients in its soymilk and tofu products." *www.vitasoy-usa.com/faqs.html*, accessed 11/23/05.

41: WestSoy website, "All of WestSoy soymilks are made with organic soymilk and certified organic by the Quality Assurance International." "Our Products" *www.westsoy.biz/products/index.html*, accessed 11/23/05.

42: Belsoy website, "FAQ," *www.belsoy.com/idbes001.htm*.

43: Sun Soy website, "The soybeans used in our products are not genetically modified." "FAQ," *www.sunsoy.com/faq.php*, accessed 11/23/05.

44: Zen Don website, Confirmed GE-Free at "Soy FAQs," *www.zendon.com*.

45: Pacific Soy websites, "The soybeans we use in each of our natural beverages are certified organic soybeans." "FAQs," *www.pacificfoods.com/products-faqs.php*.

46: Yves website, "Products," "Made with organic soy," *www.yvesveggie.com/products.php?page=1*.

47: Nancy's Cultured Soy and Dairy, "Nancy's soy is fully organic!!" "FAQs," *www.nancysyogurt.com/contact/faq.php, 11/23/05*.

48: Wholesoy website, "FAQs," "All soybeans used in products are organic." *www.wholesoycom.com/soybase.html#faq7*.

49: Stonyfield Farm website, "All Natural Cultured Soy," certified organic. *www.stonyfield.com/OurProducts/AllNaturalCulturedSoy.cfm*.

50: Soy Delicious/Turtle Mountain website, "Environmental Concerns" GMO-free to their knowledge and ability, *www.turtlemountain.com/env/gmo.html*.

51: 8th Continent website, "Our Soymilks," "Ingredients Lists," *www.8thcontinent.com/our_soymilks*.

52: Gerber products, Consumer Service representative Karla Karnemaat, "Gerber Products Company does not use genetically modified ingredients in our products. None of the fruit, vegetable, grain, dairy, or meat ingredients in our baby food products are from genetically enhanced sources. This includes our organic line of foods, Tender Harvest." 9/27/04.

53: Earth's Best, "Earth's Best is pleased to announce that on January 1, 2001 we became the first organic baby food to contain no genetically engineered ingredients (GEIs)," *www.earthsbest.com/about_eb/index.php#nogei*, accessed 10/28/05.

54: Baby's Only, confirmed organic at *www.naturesone.com/index.php*, accessed 11/18/05.

55: Beech-Nut, "We will seek to avoid the use of genetically modified ingredients wherever possible." Mary Anne Howe, Customer Service agent 10/31/05.

56: Nestlé, producer of Good Start formulas, openly uses genetically engineered soybeans and attests to their "safety and nutrition." Customer Support, 9/27/04.

57: Enfamil and Similac do not use soy protein derived from biotechnology. However, they cannot say the same for other corn/soy ingredients in the formula. In addition, neither company sources for non-rBGH milk, Enfamil and Similac Consumer Service representatives.

58: Ibid.

59: Annie's Natural, "No, we do not use GMOs and we are very thorough in our research of ingredients. We require statements from the vendors." Vicki Perham, Annie's Naturals' Customer Care, 11/17/05.

60: Braggs, labeled "certified non-GMO."

61: Spectrum has organic and nonorganic lines, some of which are third party verified with the claim "made from products that have not been genetically modified."

62: Drew's, "The things you will not find in our products are trans fats, ingredients grown from GMO seeds, artificial flavors, colors or preservatives." *www. chefdrew.com*, accessed 10/28/05.

63: Annie's Natural, "No, we do not use GMOs and we are very thorough in our research of ingredients. We require statements from the vendors." Vicki Perham, Annie's Naturals' Customer Care, 11/17/05.

64: VitaSoy, "FAQs," "Vitasoy USA uses only non-GMO ingredients in its soymilk and tofu products." *www.vitasoy-usa.com/faqs.html*, accessed 11/23/05.

65: Maranatha, "We only use third party certified organic ingredients in our certified organic foods and we request GMO-free ingredients from all suppliers." *www.nspiredfoods.com/faq.html#maranatha*, accessed 11/23/05.

66: SoyNut Butter, "All of the soybeans in I.M. Health™ SoyNut Butters are guaranteed non-GMO." *www.soynutbutter.com/faq.html*, accessed 11/23/05.

67: Mazola, "Yes, we do use GMO corn," Consumer Affairs, 11/2/05.

68: Smucker's, "It is possible that some of our products may contain ingredients derived from biotechnology." Customer Service representative, 11/2/05.

69: ConAgra Foods, "We use only ingredients that are fully approved by the USDA and the FDA." ConAgra Foods Consumer Affairs, 9/24/04.

70: ConAgra Foods, "We use only ingredients that are fully approved by the USDA and the FDA." ConAgra Foods Consumer Affairs, 9/24/04.

71: Heinz, "We seek to avoid ingredients from genetically modified sources. For example, in the case of tomatoes, we only use those bred utilizing traditional breeding technology. Additionally, we are working with non-tomato ingredient suppliers to understand the source of these ingredients and the future of the supply." Heinz Consumer Resource Center, 9/29/05.

72: Unilever, "Unilever companies are free to use ingredients derived from modified crops which have been approved by the regulatory authorities and our own clearance procedures for quality and acceptability." From *www.unilever. com/ourvalues/environmentandsociety/issues/gmos.asp*, accessed 11/2/05.

73: Kraft, "Taking these considerations into account, we currently allow the use of biotech ingredients in our products when: There is a reputable scientific consensus that the ingredient is safe; products that contain the ingredient are intended for sale only in areas where we believe they are generally acceptable to our consumers and trade customers; the ingredient is compatible with our product needs and distribution systems; using the ingredient is permitted by national regulatory authorities and no special labeling is required on the finished product." *www.kraft.com/responsibility/quality_food_biotechnology.aspx*, accessed 11/2/05.

74: Del Monte, "Our principle ingredients are not genetically modified. Anything that may be added, it is very hard for us to know." Customer Affairs representative, 11/3/05.

75: Unilever, "Unilever companies are free to use ingredients derived from modified crops which have been approved by the regulatory authorities and our own clearance procedures for quality and acceptability." From *www.unilever. com/ourvalues/environmentandsociety/issues/gmos.asp*, accessed 11/2/05.

76: Smucker's, "It is possible that some of our products may contain ingredients derived from biotechnology." Customer Service representative, 11/2/05.

77: Unilever, "Unilever companies are free to use ingredients derived from modified crops which have been approved by the regulatory authorities and our own clearance procedures for quality and acceptability." From *www.unilever. com/ourvalues/environmentandsociety/issues/gmos.asp*, accessed 11/2/05.

78: ConAgra Foods, "We use only ingredients that are fully approved by the USDA and the FDA." ConAgra Foods Consumer Affairs, 9/24/04.

79: Imagine Natural, "All nine varieties are non-GMO." *www.imaginefoods. com/pages/products/soupbroth.php*, accessed on 11/17/05.

80: Amy's Kitchen, "Amy's is made from… no GMOs." Amy's Kitchen Website, *www.amyskitchen.com/products/index.php*, accessed 10/27/05.

81: Fantastic Foods, Fantastic Foods "focuses on assuring that our agricultural crops and agricultural commodities will be from non-GMO stocks." Fantastic Foods Public Relations, 9/27/04.

82: Hain Celestial Group, "Q & A," "All products are GE-free and labeled as such (GEI-free)," *www.hainpuresnax.com/qa/index.php*, accessed 11/21/05.

83: Campbell's/Pepperidge Farm, Pepperidge Farm Web Team, "The current U.S. supply of corn and soybeans includes a mix of genetically and non-genetically modified crops. Pepperidge Farm's use of genetically modified ingredients is restricted primarily to this supply of corn and soybeans." 11/1/05.

84: Hormel, "Hormel Foods will, therefore, continue to support the crop and vegetable industries." Consumer Response Specialist for Hormel Foods, 9/17/04.

85: General Mills, "Because of the growing use of biotechnology by farmers and the way that grain gets commingled in storage and shipment, it's certainly possible that some of our products may contain ingredients that have been improved through biotechnology." Jenny Path, General Mills Consumer Services, 11/7/05.

86: ConAgra Foods, "We use only ingredients that are fully approved by the USDA and the FDA." ConAgra Foods Consumer Affairs, 9/24/04.

87: Annie's Natural, "No, we do not use GMOs and we are very thorough in our research of ingredients. We require statements from the vendors." Vicki Perham, Annie's Naturals' Customer Care, 11/ 17/05.

88: Unilever, "Unilever companies are free to use ingredients derived from modified crops which have been approved by the regulatory authorities and our own clearance procedures for quality and acceptability." From *www.unilever. com/ourvalues/environmentandsociety/issues/gmos.asp*, accessed 11/2/05.

89: Campbell's/Pepperidge Farm, Pepperidge Farm Web Team, "The current U.S. supply of corn and soybeans includes a mix of genetically and non-genetically modified crops. Pepperidge Farm's use of genetically modified ingredients is restricted primarily to this supply of corn and soybeans." 11/1/05.

90: Heinz, "We seek to avoid ingredients from genetically modified sources. For example, in the case of tomatoes, we only use those bred utilizing traditional breeding technology. Additionally, we are working with non-tomato ingredient suppliers to understand the source of these ingredients and the future of the supply." Heinz Consumer Resource Center, 9/29/05.

91: Unilever, "Unilever companies are free to use ingredients derived from modified crops which have been approved by the regulatory authorities and our own clearance procedures for quality and acceptability." From *www.unilever. com/ourvalues/environmentandsociety/issues/gmos.asp*, accessed 11/2/05.

92: ConAgra Foods, "We use only ingredients that are fully approved by the USDA and the FDA." ConAgra Foods Consumer Affairs, 9/24/04.

93: ConAgra Foods, "We use only ingredients that are fully approved by the USDA and the FDA." ConAgra Foods Consumer Affairs, 9/24/04.

94: Del Monte, "Our principle ingredients are not genetically modified. Anything that may be added, it is very hard for us to know." Customer Affairs representative, 11/3/05.

95: Hormel, "Hormel Foods will, therefore, continue to support the crop and vegetable industries." Consumer Response Specialist for Hormel Foods, 9/17/04.

96: General Mills, "Because of the growing use of biotechnology by farmers and the way that grain gets commingled in storage and shipment, it's certainly possible that some of our products may contain ingredients that have been improved through biotechnology." Jenny Path, General Mills Consumer Services, 11/7/05.

98: Amy's Kitchen, "Amy's is made from… no GMOs." Amy's Kitchen website, *www.amyskitchen.com/products/index.php*, accessed 10/27/05.

99: Annie's Natural, "No, we do not use GMOs and we are very thorough in our research of ingredients. We require statements from the vendors." Vicki Perham, Annie's Naturals' Customer Care, 11/17/05.

100: Hain Celestial Group, "Q & A," "All products are GE-free and labeled as such (GEI-free)," *www.hainpuresnax.com/qa/index.php*, accessed 11/21/05.

101: ConAgra Foods, "We use only ingredients that are fully approved by the USDA and the FDA." ConAgra Foods Consumer Affairs, 9/24/04.

102: Hormel, "Hormel Foods will, therefore, continue to support the crop and vegetable industries." Consumer Response specialist for Hormel Foods, 9/17/04.

103: Campbell's "The current U.S. supply of corn and soybeans includes a mix of genetically and non-genetically modified crops." Customer Service, 11/1/05.

104: Linda McCartney's, "Our all-natural pizzas and entrées contain no genetically modified organisms." *www.linda-mccartney.com*, 11/3/05.

105: Barbara's Bakery, Inc, "At present there are some ingredients that we cannot guarantee are GMO-free, nor can we source them either due to cost or availability." Susan Emblen-Richtsmeier, Customer Relations administrator, 10/27/05.

106: Cascadian Farms, "Why Go Organic?" *www.cfarm.com/cfarm/organic/default.aspx*, accessed 10/28/05.

107: Amy's Kitchen, "Amy's is made from… no GMOs." Amy's Kitchen website, *www.amyskitchen.com/products/index.php*, accessed 10/27/05.

108: A.C. LaRocco Pizza Company, LaRocco Pizza's "are all GMO-free." Customer Service, 10/14/04.

109: Cedarlane, "We do not use any GMOs." Customer Relations representative, 11/3/05.

110: Kraft, "Taking these considerations into account, we currently allow the use of biotech ingredients in our products when: There is a reputable scientific consensus that the ingredient is safe; products that contain the ingredient are intended for sale only in areas where we believe they are generally acceptable to our consumers and trade customers; the ingredient is compatible with our product needs and distribution systems; using the ingredient is permitted by national regulatory authorities and no special labeling is required on the finished product." From website, *www.kraft.com/responsibility/quality_food_biotechnology.aspx*, accessed 11/2/05.

111: Pinnacle Foods, "We do not exclude bioengineered ingredients in any of our products." Darlene Peters, Consumer Response representative, 11/3/05.

112: Smucker's, "It is possible that some of our products may contain ingredients derived from biotechnology." Customer Service representative, 11/2/05.

113: Campbell's "The current U.S. supply of corn and soybeans include a mix of genetically and non-genetically modified crops." Customer Service, 11/1/05.

114: Nestlé, "Gene Technology." "Nestlé supports a responsible application of gene technology for food production." *www.nestle.com/Our_Responsibility/Gene_Technology/Gene+Technology.htm*, accessed 11/1/05.

115: Nestlé, "Gene Technology." "Nestlé supports a responsible application of gene technology for food production." *www.nestle.com/Our_Responsibility/Gene_Technology/Gene+Technology.htm*, accessed 11/1/05.

116: Unilever, "Unilever companies are free to use ingredients derived from modified crops which have been approved by the regulatory authorities and our own clearance procedures for quality and acceptability." From *www.unilever.com/ourvalues/environmentandsociety/issues/gmos.asp*, accessed 11/2/05.

117: General Mills, "Because of the growing use of biotechnology by farmers and the way that grain gets commingled in storage and shipment, it's certainly possible that some of our products may contain ingredients that have been improved through biotechnology." Jenny Path, General Mills Consumer Services, 11/7/05.

118: Kellogg, "Like most other food makers in the nation, Kellogg buys the ingredients for our foods on the open market. It is likely, therefore, that all U.S. foods using these ingredients could have biotech content in the same proportion that it occurs in the national supply." From U.S. position statement on biotechnology.

119: ConAgra Foods, "We use only ingredients that are fully approved by the USDA and the FDA." ConAgra Foods Consumer Affairs, 9/24/04.

120: ConAgra Foods, "We use only ingredients that are fully approved by the USDA and the FDA." ConAgra Foods Consumer Affairs, 9/24/04.

121: Nestlé, "Gene Technology." "Nestlé supports a responsible application of gene technology for food production." *www.nestle.com/Our_Responsibility/Gene_Technology/Gene+Technology.htm*, accessed 11/1/05.

122: ConAgra Foods, "We use only ingredients that are fully approved by the USDA and the FDA." ConAgra Foods Consumer Affairs, 9/24/04.

123: Kellogg, "Like most other food makers in the nation, Kellogg buys the ingredients for our foods on the open market. It is likely, therefore, that all U.S. foods using these ingredients could have biotech content in the same proportion that it occurs in the national supply." From U.S. position statement on biotechnology.

124: Kraft, "Taking these considerations into account, we currently allow the use of biotech ingredients in our products when: There is a reputable scientific consensus that the ingredient is safe; products that contain the ingredient are intended for sale only in areas where we believe they are generally acceptable to our consumers and trade customers; the ingredient is compatible with our product needs and distribution systems; using the ingredient is permitted by national regulatory authorities and no special labeling is required on the finished product." From website, *www.kraft.com/responsibility/quality_food_biotechnology.aspx*, accessed 11/2/05.

125: Gardenburger, "We cannot guarantee that our products are non-GMO." Linda Olsen, Consumer Affairs coordinator for Gardenburger Authentic Foods Company, 10/6/05.

126: Heinz, "We seek to avoid ingredients from genetically modified sources. For example, in the case of tomatoes, we only use those bred utilizing traditional breeding technology. Additionally, we are working with non-tomato ingredient suppliers to understand the source of these ingredients and the future of the supply." Heinz Consumer Resource Center, 9/29/05.

127: ConAgra Foods, "We use only ingredients that are fully approved by the USDA and the FDA." ConAgra Foods Consumer Affairs, 9/24/04.

128: Annie's Natural, "No, we do not use GMOs and we are very thorough in our research of ingredients. We require statements from the vendors." Vicki Perham, Annie's Naturals' Customer Care, 11/7/05.

129: Lundberg Family Farms, "Lundberg Family Farms does not: Purchase GMO ingredients for their products" *www.lundberg.com/farming/gmos.shtml*, accessed 11/15/05.

130: Hain Celestial Group, "Q & A," "All products are GE-free and labeled as such (GEI-free)," *www.hainpuresnax.com/qa/index.php*, accessed 11/21/05.

131: Fantastic Foods, Fantastic Foods "focuses on assuring that our agricultural crops and agricultural commodities will be from non-GMO stocks." Fantastic Foods Public Relations, 9/27/04.

132: Amy's Kitchen, "Amy's is made from… no GMOs." Amy's Kitchen website, *www.amyskitchen.com/products/index.php*, accessed 10/27/05.

133: Kraft, "Taking these considerations into account, we currently allow the use of biotech ingredients in our products when: There is a reputable scientific consensus that the ingredient is safe; products that contain the ingredient are intended for sale only in areas where we believe they are generally acceptable to our consumers and trade customers; the ingredient is compatible with our product needs and distribution systems; using the ingredient is permitted by national regulatory authorities and no special labeling is required on the finished product." From website, *www.kraft.com/responsibility/quality_food_biotechnology.aspx*, accessed 11/2/05.

134: General Mills, "Because of the growing use of biotechnology by farmers and the way that grain gets commingled in storage and shipment, it's certainly possible that some of our products may contain ingredients that have been improved through biotechnology." Jenny Path, General Mills Consumer Services, 11/7/05.

135: Unilever, "Unilever companies are free to use ingredients derived from modified crops which have been approved by the regulatory authorities and our own clearance procedures for quality and acceptability." From *www.unilever.com/ourvalues/environmentandsociety/issues/gmos.asp*, accessed 11/2/05.

136: Quaker, "There is a high probability that some of Quaker's products contain foods developed through biotechnology." Statement from Quaker Oats Company Customer Service, 9/23/04.

137: Unilever, "Unilever companies are free to use ingredients derived from modified crops which have been approved by the regulatory authorities and our own clearance procedures for quality and acceptability." From *www.unilever.com/ourvalues/environmentandsociety/issues/gmos.asp*, accessed 11/2/05.

138: Quaker, "There is a high probability that some of Quaker's products contain foods developed through biotechnology." Statement from Quaker Oats Company Customer Service, 9/23/04.

139: Alvarado Street Bakery, "Alvarado Street Bakery would never knowingly use any ingredient (including our soy-based lecithin and organic corn) that has been genetically altered." *www.alvaradostreetbakery.com/faq_asb.html#2*, accessed 11/23/05.

140: Garden of Eatin', Hain Celestial Group, "Q & A," "All products are GE-free and labeled as such (GEI-free)," *www.hainpuresnax.com/qa/index.php*, accessed 11/21/05.

141: Interstate Brands, Consumer Affairs representative Greg Jost, "The [ingredient] specifications do not however stipulate source of ingredients in terms of geographic location, cultivation method, i.e., organic/non-organic, or seed variety identity." 11/3/05.

142: Campbell's/Pepperidge Farm, Pepperidge Farm Web Team, "The current U.S. supply of corn and soybeans includes a mix of genetically and non-genetically modified crops. Pepperidge Farm's use of genetically modified ingredients is restricted primarily to this supply of corn and soybeans." 11/1/05.

143: George Weston Bakeries/Thomas's, Consumer Relations assistant Toby Arrow, " George Weston Bakeries uses only approved ingredients conforming to health, safety, and quality assurance standards set by U.S. government and other governmental bodies worldwide. These ingredients include some that may have been derived from genetically-modified corn, soybeans, and canola." 11/2/05.

144: Bob's Red Mill, Customer Service representative, "Our products are all identity preserved. That means that the seed that was planted for the plants which yielded the grain originated from a non-GMO source." 11/2/05.

145: Rumford Baking Powder, "Rumford Baking Powder Ingredient List: Food-Grade Cornstarch (Non-GMO 'not genetically modified')" *www.yankeegrocery.com/rumford_baking.html*, accessed 11/23/05.

146: Pinnacle Foods, "We do not exclude bioengineered ingredients in any of our products." Darlene Peters, Consumer Response representative, 11/3/05.

147: General Mills, "Because of the growing use of biotechnology by farmers and the way that grain gets commingled in storage and shipment, it's certainly possible that some of our products may contain ingredients that have been improved through biotechnology." Jenny Path, General Mills Consumer Services, 11/7/05.

148: Smucker's, "It is possible that some of our products may contain ingredients derived from biotechnology." Customer Service representative, 11/2/05.

149: Pinnacle Foods, "We do not exclude bioengineered ingredients in any of our products." Darlene Peters, Consumer Response representative, 11/3/05.

150: Kraft, "Taking these considerations into account, we currently allow the use of biotech ingredients in our products when: There is a reputable scientific consensus that the ingredient is safe; products that contain the ingredient are intended for sale only in areas where we believe they are generally acceptable to our consumers and trade customers; the ingredient is compatible with our product needs and distribution systems; using the ingredient is permitted by national regulatory authorities and no special labeling is required on the finished product." From website, *www.kraft.com/responsibility/quality_food_biotechnology.aspx*, accessed 11/2/05.

151: Smucker's, "It is possible that some of our products may contain ingredients derived from biotechnology. "Customer Service representative, 11/2/05.

152: Barbara's Bakery Inc., regarding non-certified organic line, "At present there are some ingredients that we cannot guarantee are GMO-free, nor can we source them either due to cost or availability." From Susan Emblen-Richtsmeier, Customer Relations administrator, 10/27/05.

153: Health Valley, "Why Natural Foods?" "We are committed to developing and selling products that are free of genetically engineered ingredients," *www.healthvalley.com/info/why_nf.php*, accessed 11/23/05.

154: EnviroKidz Cereals, certified organic, *www.envirokidz.com/home*, accessed 11/23/05.

155: Nature's Path, certified organic, *www.naturespath.com/organics/gmos*, accessed 10/25/05.

156: Peace Cereal, "Peace Cereal has taken a strong stand against these practices, and wherever possible we have used suppliers that adhere strictly to non-GMO production methods," "Organic and Natural Ingredients," *www.peacecereal.com/Organic/OrganicAndNatural.html#GMOs*, accessed 11/23/05.

157: Cascadian Farms, "Why Go Organic?" *www.cfarm.com/cfarm/organic/default.aspx*, accessed 10/28/05.

158: General Mills, "Because of the growing use of biotechnology by farmers and the way that grain gets commingled in storage and shipment, it's certainly possible that some of our products may contain ingredients that have been improved through biotechnology." Jenny Path, General Mills Consumer Services, 11/7/05.

159: Kellogg, "Like most other food makers in the nation, Kellogg buys the ingredients for our foods on the open market. It is likely, therefore, that all U.S. foods using these ingredients could have biotech content in the same proportion that it occurs in the national supply." From U.S. position statement on biotechnology.

160: Quaker, "There is a high probability that some of Quaker's products contain foods developed through biotechnology." Statement from Quaker Oats Company Customer Service, 9/23/04.

161: Kraft, "Taking these considerations into account, we currently allow the use of biotech ingredients in our products when: There is a reputable scientific consensus that the ingredient is safe; products that contain the ingredient are intended for sale only in areas where we believe they are generally acceptable to our consumers and trade customers; the ingredient is compatible with our product needs and distribution systems; using the ingredient is permitted by national regulatory authorities and no special labeling is required on the finished product ." From website, *www.kraft.com/responsibility/quality_food_bio-technology.aspx*, accessed 11/2/05.

162: Garden of Eatin', "About Garden of Eatin'" "Our goal as a company is to produce natural and organic products without the use of genetically engineered ingredients (GEIs)," *www.gardenofeatin.com/about_us/about_goe.php*, accessed 11/21/05.

163: Hain Celestial Group, "Q & A," "All products are GE-free and labeled as such (GEI-free)," *www.hainpuresnax.com/qa/index.php*, ed 11/21/05.

164: Kettle Foods, "All of our potatoes and all of our cooking oil are non-GMO. Many Kettle™ brand products are certified organic, and thus do not contain any GMOs." "Frequently Asked Questions," *www.kettlefoods.com/index.php?cID=88*, accessed 10/ 25/05.

165: Newman's Own Organics and Newman's Own, "The soybean oil distributor for the salad dressings will not provide GE information, all other foods are GE-free." Customer Service representative from Newman's Own, 10/25/05.

166: Hain Celestial Group, "Q & A," "All products are GE-free and labeled as such (GEI-free)," *www.hainpuresnax.com/qa/index.php*, accessed 11/21/05.

167: Health Valley, "We are committed to developing and selling products that are free of genetically engineered ingredients." "Why Natural Foods?" *www.healthvalley.com/info/why_nf.php*, accessed 10/26/05.

168: Kraft, "Taking these considerations into account, we currently allow the use of biotech ingredients in our products when: There is a reputable scientific consensus that the ingredient is safe; products that contain the ingredient are intended for sale only in areas where we believe they are generally acceptable to our consumers and trade customers; the ingredient is compatible with our product needs and distribution systems; using the ingredient is permitted by national regulatory authorities and no special labeling is required on the finished product." From website, *www.kraft.com/responsibility/quality_food_bio-technology.aspx*, accessed 11/2/05.

169: Campbell's/Pepperidge Farms, Pepperidge Farm Web Team, "The current U.S. supply of corn and soybeans includes a mix of genetically and non-genetically modified crops. Pepperidge Farm's use of genetically modified ingredients is restricted primarily to this supply of corn and soybeans." 11/1/05.

170: Kellogg, "Like most other food makers in the nation, Kellogg buys the ingredients for our foods on the open market. It is likely, therefore, that all U.S. foods using these ingredients could have biotech content in the same proportion that it occurs in the national supply." From U.S. position statement on biotechnology.

171: Interstate Brands, Consumer Affairs representative Greg Jost, "The [ingredient] specifications do not however stipulate source of ingredients in terms of geographic location, cultivation method, i.e., organic/non-organic, or seed variety identity." 11/3/05.

172: Frito-Lay, "We have instructed our farmers not to grow genetically modified varieties for Frito-Lay's needs. Since we do buy some of our ingredients from outside sources, we could have genetically modified ingredients in our products." Consumer Affairs, 9/23/04.

173: Quaker, "There is a high probability that some of Quaker's products contain foods developed through biotechnology." Statement from Quaker Oats Company Customer Service, 9/23/04.

174: Pringles, "It's possible that some of the ingredients in our products may be derived from genetically modified (GM) plants." Statement from Christina at Pringles Customer Service Team, 11/9/05.

175: Clif Bar, "Our bars do not contain any genetically modified ingredients." Clif Bar Customer Service, 11/3/05.

176: Luna Bar, "Our bars do not contain any genetically modified ingredients." Clif Bar Customer Service, 11/3/05.

177: Odwalla, "Odwalla is committed to only using ingredients that were produced from crops that are not modified using modern biotechnology. We work with our suppliers to guarantee our Odwalla consumers this assurance." Statement from representative, Voice of Odwalla, 11/3/05.

178: Genisoy, "Use identity preserved, non-GMO soy, but cannot guarantee all other ingredients to be GMO-Free" 11/3/05.

179: Nestlé, "Gene Technology." "Nestlé supports a responsible application of gene technology for food production." *www.nestle.com/Our_Responsibility/Gene_Technology/Gene+Technology.htm*, accessed 11/1/05.

180: General Mills, "Because of the growing use of biotechnology by farmers and the way that grain gets commingled in storage and shipment, it's certainly possible that some of our products may contain ingredients that have been improved through biotechnology." Jenny Path, General Mills Consumer Services, 11/7/05.

181: Quaker, "There is a high probability that some of Quaker's products contain foods developed through biotechnology." Statement from Quaker Oats Company Customer Service, 9/23/04.

182: Kraft, "Taking these considerations into account, we currently allow the use of biotech ingredients in our products when: There is a reputable scientific consensus that the ingredient is safe; products that contain the ingredient are intended for sale only in areas where we believe they are generally acceptable to our consumers and trade customers; the ingredient is compatible with our product needs and distribution systems; using the ingredient is permitted by national regulatory authorities and no special labeling is required on the finished product." From website, *www.kraft.com/responsibility/quality_food_bio-technology.aspx*, accessed 11/2/05.

183: Balance Bar, "In all likelihood Balance Bar products may contain genetically engineered ingredients." Balance Bar Web Team on 10/6/05.

184: Endangered Species Chocolate, "About Our Chocolate," "All of our suppliers guarantee that the ingredients we use in the production of our chocolate, do not contain genetically modified organisms." *www.chocolatebar.com/FAQ.asp?TypeID=94&DeptID=0#3*, accessed 11/21/05.

185: Newman's Own, "The soybean oil distributor for the salad dressings will not provide GE information, all other foods are GE-free." Customer Service representative, 10/25/05.

186: Ghirardelli Chocolate, "Ghirardelli Chocolate Company will do everything possible to purchase and use raw materials that test negative for GMOs." Vicki Wong, Ghirardelli Chocolate Company Research and Development, 9/27/04.

187: Nestlé, "Gene Technology." "Nestlé supports a responsible application of gene technology for food production." *www.nestle.com/Our_Responsibility/Gene_Technology/Gene+Technology.htm*, accessed 11/1/05.

188: Hershey's, "It is possible that ingredients from common commodities, such as corn and soy, have been derived through agricultural biotechnology." Hershey's Public Affairs Department.

189: Kraft, "Taking these considerations into account, we currently allow the use of biotech ingredients in our products when: There is a reputable scientific consensus that the ingredient is safe; products that contain the ingredient are intended for sale only in areas where we believe they are generally acceptable to our consumers and trade customers; the ingredient is compatible with our product needs and distribution systems; using the ingredient is permitted by national regulatory authorities and no special labeling is required on the finished product." From website, *www.kraft.com/responsibility/quality_food_bio-*

technology.aspx, accessed 11/2/05.

190: Jelly Belly, "We were able to obtain our proprietary-blend of corn starch made from non-GM corn." Consumer Affairs representative for Jelly Belly Candy Company, 9/28/04.

191: Nestlé, "Gene Technology." "Nestlé supports a responsible application of gene technology for food production." www.nestle.com/Our_Responsibility/Gene_Technology/Gene+Technology.htm, accessed 11/1/05.

192: Kraft, "Taking these considerations into account, we currently allow the use of biotech ingredients in our products when: There is a reputable scientific consensus that the ingredient is safe; products that contain the ingredient are intended for sale only in areas where we believe they are generally acceptable to our consumers and trade customers; the ingredient is compatible with our product needs and distribution systems; using the ingredient is permitted by national regulatory authorities and no special labeling is required on the finished product." From website: www.kraft.com/responsibility/quality_food_biotechnology.aspx, accessed 11/2/05.

193: Hershey's, "It is possible that ingredients from common commodities, such as corn and soy, have been derived through agricultural biotechnology." Hershey's Public Affairs Department.

194: After the Fall, "We have established a documentation program for all of our natural products and their respective ingredients, with the ultimate goal of utilizing only ingredients grown and produced without the use of biotechnology." Statement from Diane Contreras, Smucker's Customer Relations, 11/3/05.

195: Eden, "GMO Stance." "Eden's Purchasing Department... does everything possible to make sure our food is free of GEOs". www.edenfoods.com/issues_geo.html, accessed 10/28/05

196: Cascadian Farms, "Why Go Organic?" www.cfarm.com/cfarm/organic/default.aspx, accessed 10/28/05.

197: Odwalla, "Odwalla is committed to only using ingredients that were produced from crops that are not modified using modern biotechnology. We work with our suppliers to guarantee our Odwalla consumers this assurance." Statement from representative, Voice of Odwalla, 11/3/05.

198: Coca-Cola, "Biotech corn is used in combination with traditional varieties in some parts of the world to manufacture our ingredients." Industry and Consumer Affairs for the Coca-Cola Company, 10/1/04.

199: Pepsi, "Some of our ingredients are derived from botanical sources, such as corn, however the ingredients used in our products are highly purified and contain no carryover genetic material." Consumer Communication, 9/17/04.

200: Kraft, "Taking these considerations into account, we currently allow the use of biotech ingredients in our products when: There is a reputable scientific consensus that the ingredient is safe; products that contain the ingredient are intended for sale only in areas where we believe they are generally acceptable to our consumers and trade customers; the ingredient is compatible with our product needs and distribution systems; using the ingredient is permitted by national regulatory authorities and no special labeling is required on the finished product." From website, www.kraft.com/responsibility/quality_food_biotechnology.aspx, accessed 11/2/05.

201: Nestlé, "Gene Technology." "Nestlé supports a responsible application of gene technology for food production." www.nestle.com/Our_Responsibility/Gene_Technology/Gene+Technology.htm, accessed 11/1/05.

202: Blue Sky Natural, Hansen Soda "Per our Quality Control Manager, Blue Sky Natural Sodas and Hansen Soda are 'Not GMO Free.'" Karen Kinnicutt, Consumer Relations, 11/7/05.

203: Procter & Gamble, "It's possible that some of the ingredients in our products may be derived from genetically modified (GM) plants." Procter & Gamble team representative, 11/10/05.

204: Ocean Spray, "The high fructose corn syrup used to sweeten some of our products may or may not have been produced with corn that was a product of biotechnology." Ocean Spray Consumer Affairs representative, 11/14/05.

205: See www.kraft.com/responsibility/quality_food_biotechnology.aspx.

206: See www.nestleusa.com/PubFAQ/FAQs.aspx.

207: E-mail from Jenny Path, General Mills Consumer Services, November 7, 2005.

208: E-mail from Perla Salas, Kellogg's Consumer Affairs, April 19, 2005.

209: E-mail from Heinz Consumer Resource Center, September 30, 2004.

210: E-mail from Frito-Lay Consumer Affairs, September 23, 2004.

211: Letter from Rebecca Smith, manager of consumer communication, September 17, 2004.

212: E-mail from Kari Bjorhus, Consumer Affairs, April, 20 2005.

213: E-mail from ConAgra Consumer Affairs department, April, 20 2005.

214: E-mail from Campbell's Soup Customer Support, November 1, 2005.

215: E-mail from Goldie Taylor, director of communications and public affairs, September, 30 2004.

216: E-mail from Hershey's Public Affairs Department, September, 29 2004.

217: E-mail from Hormel Consumer Response Specialist, September 17, 2004.

218: See www.unilever.com/ourvalues/environmentandsociety/issues/gmos.asp.

219: Conversation with Technical Service Department, November 22, 2005, 229-225-3800.

220: Campbell's/Pepperidge Farms, Pepperidge Farm Web Team, "The current US supply of corn and soybeans includes a mix of genetically and non-genetically modified crops. Pepperidge Farm's use of genetically modified ingredients is restricted primarily to this supply of corn and soybeans." 11/1/05.

ACKNOWLEDGMENTS

Center for Food Safety

Associate Editors: Maggie Douglas, Rebecca Spector
Research and Writing: Heather Whitehead, Ellen Kittredge, Isabelle Reining, Anne Hillson, Rhodes Yepsen, Jillian Drewes, Deborah Press, Paige Beckley, Jessica Dowling, Dan Zoll
Technical Review: Doug Gurian-Sherman, Ph.D.

The Center for Food Safety is also grateful to The CornerStone Campaign for its support for this project.

COLOPHON

The main text was typeset in Perpetua, created in 1928 by Eric Gill, an English artist-craftsman known for his mastery of typography, letter cutting, sculpture and wood engraving, and in Trump Mediaeval, created by Georg Trump between 1954 and 1962. Sidebars were mostly typeset in ScalaSans, designed by Martin Majoor in 1999.

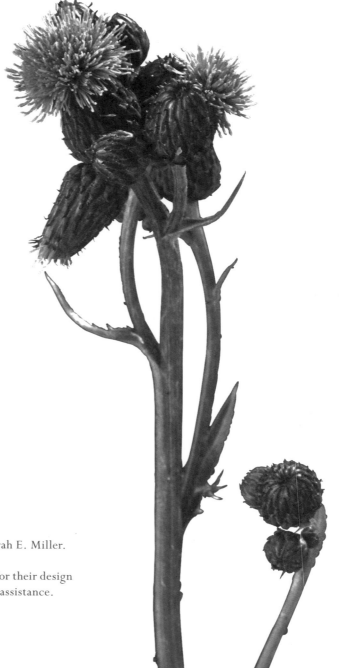

Publisher and Creative Director: Raoul Goff
Executive Directors: Michael Madden & Peter Beren
Acquisitions Editor: Raoul Goff
Art Directors: Iain Morris & Daniela Sklan
Designers: Usana Das Shadday & Sarah E. Miller
Cover & Booklet Design: Daniela Sklan
Project Editors: Emilia Thiuri, Mariah Bear & Phil Catalfo
Production Manager: Lisa Bartlett & Nam Nguyen
Studio Production: Noah Potkin

PHOTO CREDITS
Steve Cole / Getty Images: 4
Lily Films: 8 (middle right) , 24 (bottom), 27 (top), 28 (6th & 8th from left), 31 (both lower images), 33, 49, 65, 67, 68, 69 (bottom), 72 (top right), 111 (lower 4 images)
Chris Bryant: 11 (upper right), 35 (lower right), 98, 99, 100 (bottom), 108, 110 (left)
Scott Bauer: 31 (top), 60, 118
Stephen Ausmus: 40
Don Burgett: 53 (bottom)
Peggy Grebb: 55 (top)
Jered Lawson: 64 (upper left), 95, 100 (top)
Paul Bousquet: 66 (top)
Rodale Press: 66 (lower 3), 104 (top)
Zachary Griffin: 73
Maggie Hallahan: 94 and 104 (bottom)
Lower two logos on page 112 © 2005 Sonia Taylor/www.errantart.com

Additional photography provided by the USDA, Usana Das Shadday, Scott Erwert and Sarah E. Miller.

Earth Aware would also like to give a special thank you to Ian Szymkowiak and Alan Hebel for their design work, Gabriel Ely for his illustrations and Monika Lasiewski and Carina Cha for editorial assistance.